THE JARGON-BUSTER'S
GUIDE TO
HEART DISEASE

THE JARGON-BUSTER'S GUIDE TO HEART DISEASE

All you need to know
in words you can understand

DR DUNCAN DYMOND

metro

ACKNOWLEDGEMENTS

To my long-suffering family and to all my
patients and colleagues who have unwittingly
contributed to this book

First published in Great Britain in 1996
by Metro Books,
19 Gerrard Street,
London W1V 7LA

Dr Duncan Dymond is hereby identified as the author of
this work in accordance with Section 77 of the Copyright,
Designs and Patents Act 1988.

British Library Cataloguing in Publication Data.
A CIP record of this book is available on request
from the British Library.

ISBN   1 900512 00 9

10 9 8 7 6 5 4 3 2 1

Typeset by SX Composing DTP, Rayleigh, Essex
Printed in Great Britain by
Cox & Wyman Ltd, Reading, Berkshire

Diagrams by Richard Burgess

Contents

AUTHOR'S NOTE

Every profession or trade has its own mini-language or jargon. This method of communication is fine within that trade or profession, but outsiders may be muddled by the use of unfamiliar terms. Non-lawyers who have tried to make head or tail of a legal document, for example, will usually find their eyes glaze over at the endless sentences with no punctuation and full of incomprehensible terms. You could argue that it does not really matter, that life is hardly likely to be seriously affected by failing to understand the finer points of the legal process, or what on earth bankers mean when they talk about 'M3' or 'M0'.

It is somewhat different with medical matters, however. There can be nothing more uncomfortable than being a patient in a room with two or more doctors talking about you, using obscure terms and medical jargon. They are, after all, talking about your body and your illness, maybe your very survival, not some abstract prediction about the value of the pound against the yen. The use of jargon may be acceptable in medical conferences, but not for doctors explaining illnesses and treatments to their patients. Now, more than ever, patients need to understand what treatment is proposed for them, and why. They need to understand the risks and benefits of each potential treatment and what they can expect afterwards. In my experience as a heart specialist at Bart's Hospital in London, many patients' anxieties about treatments and possible complications can be avoided by careful, jargon-free explanations to the patient and their family before and after treatment. This is particularly important in the field of heart disease, where the last twenty years have seen a dramatic extension of the treatments available, often involving the use of high technology, as well as the number and type of drugs that are prescribed.

Unfortunately, the prevalence of medical jargon may act as a huge barrier towards communication, with many doctors either unwilling or unable to find the right terminology to help their patients understand what is wrong with them and what their treatment involves. In many cases this is simply due to lack of time. In others, however, doctors may simply be poor communicators or bad explainers and even resent questions from patients, believing instead that the patient should accept the offered advice with blind faith, or what I call the 'anything you say, doctor' syndrome.

People find the world of medicine fascinating. Television series such as 'Casualty' and 'Cardiac Arrest' have captured the public imagination, and one only has to scan the newspapers to come across articles on the latest medical technology. Bookshops contain numerous offerings from health and fitness experts on subjects ranging from how to look after your heart, to living with angina. Even these publications, however, may be full of jargon and assume, incorrectly, that people are familiar with basic medical concepts, and some of these books are about as user friendly as the average computer manual!

In *The Jargon-Buster's Guide to Heart Disease* I have tried to write a jargon-free, user-friendly explanation of what the heart is, how it works, what can go wrong with it and why, what treatments are available and what they consist of. This book should not be regarded as a do-it-yourself-guide to diagnosis, nor is it within the scope of the book to explain the actions and side-effects of every possible medication that heart specialists may use. The main aim of the book is to try to demystify the topic of heart disease so that the reader will become familiar with most of the common heart conditions he or she will be likely to encounter and as a result of this, be able to take an informed view of the various treatments on offer. Having said that, may I wish all readers a long, healthy and doctor-free life.

INTRODUCTION

Most people will know or be related to someone who has had a heart problem. This reflects the very high incidence of heart disease in the developed world. In Chapter 1 I will describe the various components of the heart, how they all work and what can make them go wrong.

When we talk about heart disease being the biggest single killer in the western world, we mean disease of the arteries which supply oxygen to the heart muscle. These are known as coronary arteries and it is problems with these arteries that cause so many deaths. Death rates are described by medical statisticians as the number of deaths per 100,000 of the population. For example, if the population of a country was exactly one million, and 500 people died per year of the given disease, the death rate would be described as 50 per 100,000. In the United Kingdom in 1990 there were 292 deaths per 100,000 of the population, male and female, compared with 68 per 100,000 dying of lung cancer. In other words, death from disease of the arteries of the heart was four times more common than death due to lung cancer. The death rate has fallen, slowly but steadily, from a peak in 1985, although it still ranks as the number one killer. It would be nice to think that this downward trend in death rates is due to improved medical care, new technology and better surgical skills. However, education of the population on how to prevent heart disease in the first place should be every bit as important as medical ways of dealing with the disease once it has become established. Unfortunately, this is easier said than done.

Although traditionally seen as a male disease, women are increasingly being affected. You may be surprised to know that in 1990, in women between the ages of 45 and 64, there were 97 deaths per 100,000 from coronary artery disease, and 79 per 100,000 from breast cancer. In women between 65 and 74 years of age there were four times as many deaths from coronary disease as there were from breast cancer; in women over the age of 75 the difference is nearly tenfold.

There are wide regional differences in the incidence of coronary artery disease and the number of deaths from it. Within the United Kingdom, Scotland has a particularly high incidence of coronary deaths, just as in the United States, Florida does badly. This can partly be explained by the fact that many Americans migrate to Florida in their retirement years and the incidence of deaths from coronary disease increases with age. After all, you might as well have your heart attack in the sun, as opposed to the frozen mid-west! Some of the differences between races are more difficult to explain: some Asian sub-groups have a particularly high incidence of coronary artery disease, while the Japanese have quite a low rate, and the condition is rarer in those of Afro-Caribbean origin.

The body is an amazing machine and we have not yet found it possible to design anything with as many moving parts (such as a car or an aeroplane) that can last 70, 80 years or more without falling apart. It is not just the heart that is subject to the ageing process. As we get older, our joints become less flexible, our muscles weaken, our thought processes slow and our ability to fight off infection is diminished. Arteries all over the body show signs of wear and tear as we get older, yet it is the coronary arteries which appear to be most vulnerable. This explains why heart specialists are overwhelmed with work, their clinics full and their waiting lists long. There are just not enough heart specialists in the United Kingdom to cope with the problem (in contrast with the United States where there are probably too many!). One way of making the best use of our limited resources would be if heart specialists only saw the patients they needed to see. Most specialists would agree that a large number of people who come to outpatient clinics have nothing wrong with them. Sometimes this is because the GP may not have spent enough time with the patient, preferring instead to pass the buck to the specialist, and sometimes because patients put their GPs under pressure to refer them to a specialist even if the GP thinks it unnecessary.

It is equally true, though, that there are patients with symptoms of heart disease who fail to recognise them as such and do not seek medical advice until it is too late. Even in the spring of 1996, I continue to be amazed by the level of confusion among the general public about what a heart attack actually means, and which symptoms should start alarm bells ringing and which can be safely ignored. This is not meant to be a criticism of the public, who cannot be expected to be experts in medical matters. I see it rather as a failure of both government and the medical profession to educate the public properly. The average British patient hasn't a clue what questions to ask his or her medical adviser. I contrast this with the situation in the United States, where I recall being given the third degree by a truck driver from Wisconsin, about how many procedures I had done, what my success rate was, and how many complications I had experienced over the last five years! I am not masochistic enough to wish to be subjected to this by every patient I see, but relations between patient and doctor would be a lot easier if they spoke a common language.

As an example of how jargon destroys the relationship

between doctor and patient, let me recount a two-line conversation:

DOCTOR: Well, Mr Jackson, we will implant a fixed-rate pacemaker into your heart via the cephalic vein.

PATIENT: Like hell you will!

Patient exits stage left as fast as his legs can carry him, never to be seen again.

It turned out later that the patient thought he was to have a *fifth-rate* pacemaker inserted into his heart via his *phallic* vein! No wonder he fled so quickly. I can assure male readers that the vein on their most prized possession is safe from attack by cardiologists!

There is no logical reason to expect the lay public to be familiar with terms like 'fixed-rate' and 'cephalic'. The terrified Mr Jackson would have been more at ease had the doctor concerned avoided the use of technical and anatomical jargon.

Not only can failure of communication between doctor and patient cause fear, but telling patients too little can also cause embarrassment. One example, when I was a medical student doing general surgery, springs to mind. The consultant, a kind and softly spoken man, was talking to a patient, a retired colonel, about symptoms suggestive of an enlarged prostate gland. The consultant needed to examine the prostate, which involves inserting a finger into the rectum, or back passage. The conversation went like this:

CONSULTANT: Right, sir, please get on that couch, lie on your left side and draw your knees up to your chest so I can examine your prostate gland.

The patient did as was asked. The consultant put a disposable rubber glove on his hand, smeared some lubricant jelly on his index finger, and inserted the finger into the patient's bottom.

COLONEL: How DARE you touch me there, sir!!!

With one bound the furious colonel leaped off the couch and stormed out of the room, all bristling moustache and popping eyes, leaving the consultant open-mouthed and speechless, and we students trying unsuccessfully to contain our mirth.

I hope that by the time you reach the end of this book you will not only have a better understanding of all the jargon that your GP or heart specialist might throw at you, but also have the confidence to request an explanation for anything you don't understand. If in doubt – ask!

1

JARGON-BUSTER'S GUIDE TO THE HEART

We take most of our body parts for granted. While we work, rest or play our brains control the activities of our nervous system, our stomachs and intestines work tirelessly to digest food, our livers to build up proteins and produce waste products, our kidneys to filter the waste products from the blood and produce urine and our bone marrow to produce blood cells, seven days a week, twenty-four hours a day. We tend not to be too emotionally attached to most of our organs (anyone expecting a smutty joke here will be disappointed) and most people tend not to become obsessed with their liver, stomach, intestines or kidneys. I have never come across a patient who has asked: 'Doctor, I am really worried about my spleen, could you please check it over?'

It is very different with the heart. The beating of the heart reminds us continually of its presence. We are aware of it working harder when running for a bus or climbing the stairs and we can often feel our heartbeat when lying in bed at night. Many people find it impossible to lie on their left side, because the sensation of the heartbeat transmitted through the pillow and mattress is disturbing. We perceive the heart as the one organ vital to survival.

In fact the heart is no more important than the brain or the liver, without which, of course, survival is impossible. But somehow it is thought of not only as the centre of our physical being, but also the centre of the soul, the spirit and the emotions. The *Oxford Dictionary of Quotations* contains more references to the heart than to any other part of the body. When we are miserable, we describe our hearts as being broken. Fear makes the heart race and disappointment makes it sink. Unrequited love makes our hearts ache.

If the great poets and romantic writers were to examine a heart, they would be deeply disappointed for in no way does it resemble the pink, rounded structure pierced by Cupid's arrow or as depicted on playing cards. At the risk of shattering your illusions I will try to explain the various components that make up a heart and how it works.

Most people know roughly where the heart is, namely in the chest between the neck and the stomach. Far from being confined to the left side of the chest, it is more or less central in position. It is somewhat triangular in shape with the tip of the triangle close to or just below the position of the left nipple. In conditions which force the heart to enlarge, this tip, the apex, is pushed out downwards and outwards, towards the left-hand side of the chest, in line with the left armpit. The heart is surrounded by a very thin, transparent membrane or lining, a bit like a thin polythene freezer bag. This membrane is called the *pericardium* and it protects the heart as it beats continuously, throughout our lives. Other organs in the body have similar protective linings: the lungs have the *pleura* and the intestines are protected by the *peritoneum*. The pre-fix *peri* means 'surrounding' or 'outside', as in the word periphery.

THE BODY'S ENGINE

The heart has only one purpose and that is to pump blood, which carries oxygen, around the body. This needs to be done in order to deliver a continuous supply of oxygen to all the organs and structures of the body, and to clear away the waste materials the organs and tissues produce. The heart can be compared to a pump in a central heating system. When this pump is activated, hot water flows around the house into the radiators and gives off its heat which warms the rooms, just as blood flowing into an organ gives up oxygen to keep the tissues alive.

Water that is passed through the radiator needs to be returned to the boiler for reheating before it is sent around again. Similarly, blood that has given up its oxygen must return to the heart in order for a fresh supply of oxygen to be taken on board and to be pumped around the body again. To this end, the heart and the lungs work together closely. When we breathe in, oxygen is extracted from the air and passes from the lungs into the blood. When we breathe out, the air contains a gas called carbon dioxide which is one of the waste materials produced by the body's activities. The carbon dioxide that we breathe out is at a body temperature of 37°C, which is why on cold mornings our breath looks like steam.

Different parts of the body need more or less oxygen at different times. The circulation in our bodies automatically diverts blood to areas that need more oxygen at the expense of other areas that may not need so much. For example, during physical exercise the body automatically diverts blood away from the stomach and intestines to give more oxygen to the muscles of the legs and arms. Conversely, after a meal, blood will be diverted from the muscles which we normally use while jogging to increase the flow through the digestive system. Our grandmothers who would not allow us to rush around after a meal may not have known much about the circulation, but they gave good advice. Using the central heating analogy again, many modern systems have radiators with individual thermostats, so if a floor of a house or particular room is not being used, the thermostat can be turned down so that hot water does not go to that particular radiator and heat the room unnecessarily. Although this is done to save money on fuel rather than out of need, the principle is the same.

Given that the job of the heart is to pump blood around the body, it follows that the bulk of the heart consists of muscle. The contraction of the heart muscle expels the blood into the circulation and the wave produced by the contraction produces the pulse you feel in your wrist. Between contractions, the heart muscle needs to relax in order to fill up for the next beat. The heart muscle is known by doctors as the *myocardium*, *myo* meaning muscle and *cardium* meaning heart.

In order to understand how a muscle works, by contracting and relaxing, you can look at how your biceps muscle works on the front of your arm. Place the fingers of your right hand on the front of your left upper arm and bend your left elbow. You will feel the muscle tense as it contracts and as the attachments at the elbow joint pull the forearm up towards the shoulder. Now let your arm straighten again, and you will feel the muscle becoming less tense as it relaxes. If you now repeatedly bend and straighten the elbow, you will have an idea of how the heart muscle contracts and relaxes continuously throughout our lifetime.

The major difference between the biceps and other limb muscles and the muscle of the heart is that the heart contracts and relaxes whether you tell it to or not, in other words, it is involuntary. There are stories of fakirs who have perfected the power of self-control and are able to slow their heartbeat down at will, but we mere mortals who are more worried about our mortgages than meditation should be content to let our hearts get on with it! The jargon for the contraction phase of the heart is *systole* (pronounced sis-to-lee) and the relaxation phase is called *diastole* (pronounced dye-as-to-lee). You may have come across these words in relation to blood pressure readings. Blood pressure is usually given as two numbers, a top one called *systolic*, and a bottom one called *diastolic*. These terms refer to the pressure in the arteries of the body when the heart is contracting and relaxing respectively.

Although it looks boring from the outside, if one imagines the heart opening like a book it becomes more interesting. It consists of four chambers. The two upper chambers, each called an *atrium*, act as filling chambers for the blood coming back into the heart. The word atrium has been borrowed by large hotels to describe the main lobby where people collect. The two lower chambers are each known as a *ventricle* and these chambers are the main pumps of the heart. There is a right and a left atrium and a right and a left ventricle (this means your own right and left, not as you look at a diagram of the heart). You might wonder why I am going into such detailed description of the structure of the heart, but if any of you, your friends or relatives have been told you are suffering from 'atrial this' or 'ventricular that', at least these terms will now have some meaning. So I make no apologies for taking you on this journey through the heart and explaining some of the technical words that may be used.

In normal circumstances, each of the heart's four chambers is separated from its neighbour. The right-side chambers are separated from those on the left by a structure called the *septum*. This can be regarded as a type of wall and, as you will see shortly, it prevents blood which has given up its oxygen with mixing from blood that contains oxygen. Defects in the septum can either be present at birth (called *congenital defects*) or in some cases can be acquired as a result of damage to the heart in later life.

In order for the heart to work efficiently, there is a system of valves which open and shut at the right time to allow blood to pass from one chamber to the next and to permit blood to flow in one direction only. The valves of the heart can be regarded as doors to a room; one door lets you into the room and another lets you out. In the heart the valves prevent blood from going the wrong way, or leaking back from where it has just come from. An inlet valve separates the upper chamber from the lower chamber on each side. They open to let the blood pass from the upper chambers to the lower chambers and close when the lower chambers contract to expel the blood into the circulation, so that blood can't leak backwards. A right and a left outlet valve open when the heart pumps to let blood into the circulation and they shut during the filling phase between heartbeats.

A JOURNEY THROUGH THE HEART

So how is the blood routed through the heart and lungs? A sensible place to start is with the right-side upper chamber (*right atrium*) as shown in the diagram overleaf. This chamber collects all the blood that needs to come back into the heart once it has given up its oxygen to the organs and tissues of the body. The blood drains towards the heart through a collection of veins. The veins all join together to form larger veins which eventually enter the right atrium through two enormous veins, each called a *vena cava*. One enters the top and the other the bottom of the right atrium. The upper vena cava is called the superior , and the lower the inferior. (Superior and inferior mean upper and lower, and have nothing to do with social class or quality!)

When the right atrium is full of blood it contracts, blood passes through the inlet valve into the right-side pumping chamber (*right ventricle*) and about a fifth of a second later this ventricle contracts. At this point the inlet valve shuts and the outlet valve opens to allow blood to pass out of the

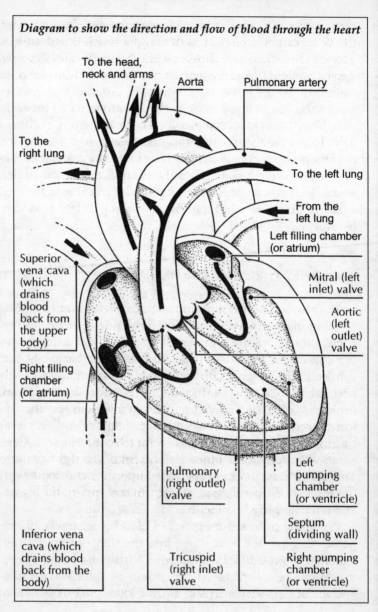

Diagram to show the direction and flow of blood through the heart

To the head, neck and arms

Aorta

Pulmonary artery

To the right lung

To the left lung

From the left lung

Left filling chamber (or atrium)

Superior vena cava (which drains blood back from the upper body)

Mitral (left inlet) valve

Aortic (left outlet) valve

Right filling chamber (or atrium)

Pulmonary (right outlet) valve

Left pumping chamber (or ventricle)

Septum (dividing wall)

Inferior vena cava (which drains blood back from the body)

Tricuspid (right inlet) valve

Right pumping chamber (or ventricle)

right side of the heart into a large tube which divides into two and carries blood into the right and left lung respectively. This tube which leaves the heart is called the *pulmonary artery* (pulmonary being the technical word for lung).

In the lungs, the blood gives off carbon dioxide, which we breathe out, and takes oxygen on board. From the lungs, the blood then flows through *pulmonary veins* into the left-side upper or filling chamber (*left atrium*), with a replenished oxygen supply. The left-side inlet valve then opens into the left-side pumping chamber of the heart (*left ventricle*). When the left ventricle contracts, the left inlet valve shuts and blood is pumped out through the outlet valve of the left ventricle into an extremely large artery called the *aorta*, which is the main artery of the body. The left ventricle is thought of as the main pump as it has responsibility for the whole body. It is more important than the right ventricle, has more work to do, and is therefore much thicker. All the right ventricle has to do is to pump blood through the lungs and that does not require much work.

Although the course of events I have described is how you would see things if you were a blood cell, in reality the two upper chambers (atria) contract at the same time and the two lower chambers (ventricles) together, about a fifth of a second later. This very short delay makes the heart action efficient and allows the atria to empty their contents into the ventricles immediately prior to the ventricles expelling the blood towards the lungs or around the body. When disorders of the cardiac rhythm occur the heart's pump becomes less efficient.

ARTERIES AND VEINS

People are often confused by the difference between an

artery and a *vein*. The difference is simply that arteries take blood out of the heart and veins bring it back. An analogy can be drawn again with the central heating pump in a house which pumps hot water to the radiators; the pipe leading into the pump for the radiators can be regarded as a vein and that which leaves the pump is like an artery.

The most obvious place to find a vein is at the back of your hand or at your elbow. A vein is where a doctor might insert a needle to take blood for a sample, or to put a drip up if he needs to give you intravenous fluids. They are thin-walled bluey-green structures.

The aorta, the main artery leaving the heart with oxy-genated blood, can be regarded as the trunk of a tree, and in medicine we often refer to *'the arterial tree'*. Just as the trunk of a tree gives off boughs, which in turn give off branches, then smaller branches and twigs, so the aorta gives off big branches which supply the head and neck, and then the arms. It turns downwards into the abdomen where it gives off further branches to the stomach, intestines, kidneys etc. In the lower part of the abdomen the aorta divides into two arteries, one going down to each leg. Small branches, too numerous to name are given off throughout the whole course of the aorta. Every organ, be it ever so small (yes, even *that* one) has its own arterial supply.

When a stone is dropped into a pond, it produces waves or ripples that spread out from the centre. In the same way, the contraction of the heart produces a wave that can be felt at strategic points around the body. This is called a *pulse*. Many people think that the only point a pulse is felt is at the wrist and most readers will be familiar with how to take their wrist pulse just below the base of the thumb. In normal circumstances the number of beats per minute at the wrist tells you exactly how fast your heart is beating. Doctors can feel pulses wherever the arteries are close to the surface. A pulse can be felt on both sides of the neck from the *carotid* artery, which conducts blood up into the brain, or near the skin crease in each groin, where the *femoral* arteries take blood into the legs. Sometimes (although with more difficulty), pulses can be taken on the back of the knee, and there are two pulses on each foot; one on the front of the foot, in the middle of the instep, the other just behind the inner ankle bone. Your doctor can learn a lot about the state of your heart by the character of the pulse.

Going back to the hand, you will feel the pulse at your wrist and see the veins on the back of your hand, but the real business happens between the artery you can feel and the veins you can see. The artery divides up into smaller and smaller branches, eventually becoming too small to be seen by the naked eye. These are called *capillaries*. If you look at your finger nails, they are normally quite pink. If you press on a nail, you can make it go white and when you release the pressure it becomes pink again. This is because you are squeezing the capillaries; it is this fine capillary network that makes our skin look pink and healthy. The capillaries are in direct contact with the tissues and give them oxygen. When they have given up their oxygen and collected the waste products they join up to tiny veins, which then join together to join the big veins, which you can see. You will notice that the veins do not pulsate, and this is because the energy delivered by each heartbeat has been dissipated in conducting the blood through the arterial tree into the capillaries, so by the time it gets into the veins there are no ripples left.

The capillaries in the skin are quite sensitive to heat, or lack of it. In hot weather, when our body temperature is high, we need to lose more heat. Unlike dogs we do not have to sit with our tongues hanging out to lose body heat, but the capillaries in the skin open up and transfer heat from our bodies into the atmosphere. Similarly, when we are cold and need to conserve heat, the capillaries in the skin shut down and that is why our hands may look white or even bluish in cold weather. Some people find their hands and feet are always cold and this is often put down to 'poor circulation'. Their arteries and veins are usually all intact, however; they may just have sensitive capillaries and their hands and feet are always cold. But it does not mean that they have bad circulation. Remember that next time your sleeping partner's feet feel like two blocks of ice even in high summer! The adage 'cold hands, warm heart' is not necessarily inaccurate.

So how does the blood get back to the heart? We don't have pumps in our hands and feet to pump the blood back but there are several complicated mechanisms for returning the blood to the heart. These include gravity (in the case of the head and the neck), the contraction of the muscles (particularly in the case of the legs) and also the act of breathing in actually sucks blood back into the chest, in the same way that opening a pair of bellows sucks air in.

FUEL PIPES, WIRING AND BATTERY

So far I have not mentioned how the heart receives its own blood supply to keep the muscle working, or how the heart knows how fast to beat. Like any of the muscles in the arms, legs, chest or abdomen, the heart needs an adequate blood supply. Immediately above the outlet valve of the left pumping chamber (ventricle), two arteries arise from the main arterial trunk (aorta) and turn back on themselves to deliver blood into the heart muscle These arteries are called the *coronary arteries* and are shown in the diagram on page 22. They are called coronary arteries because the early anatomists who described them were lyrical individuals and they thought the arteries lay on the surface of the heart rather like a coronet sits on the head!

Blood full of oxygen passes down the coronary arteries and there is a system of capillaries and veins in the heart in the same way as in other organs. The right coronary artery gives off a few branches which supply the right pumping chamber (ventricle), but most of the blood goes to supplying the floor and back wall of the left ventricle, which, as we have seen, has much more work to do. The left coronary artery divides almost immediately into two arteries; one which runs down the front of the heart and one which runs down the back.

I have mentioned before that, unlike other muscles, the heart muscle contracts and beats without being consciously told to do so. Every muscle in the body has a nerve supply. Messages which tell the muscle to contract are conveyed by electrical currents which pass down those nerves. If the nerves are damaged anywhere in their course the muscles cannot contract. All of us will have banged our elbow exactly where the nerve lies – often called the funny bone but the sensation in your arm is hardly funny. Similarly, if we sit cross-legged too long we get pins and needles, and find it difficult to walk. This is because we have been pressing on the nerve to the leg.

The heart also needs electrical signals to make it beat, and can be thought of as having its own electrical wiring system which sends messages to the heart to contract. These impulses originate in the heart's 'battery' which lies in the right filling chamber (atrium). It is really an amazing structure, called the *sinus node*. Although not perceptible to the naked eye this battery sends out electrical impulses which may keep the heart beating for 80 years or more. However convincing television advertisements may be, none of the manufacturers of commercial batteries can compete with this! If the heart's battery discharges an

Diagram of the outside of the heart viewed from the front, showing the most important arteries and veins

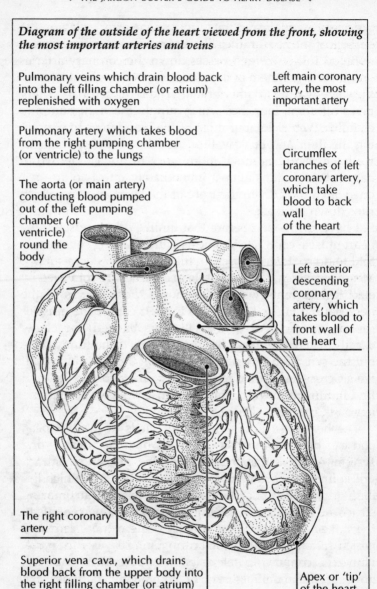

Pulmonary veins which drain blood back into the left filling chamber (or atrium) replenished with oxygen

Left main coronary artery, the most important artery

Pulmonary artery which takes blood from the right pumping chamber (or ventricle) to the lungs

Circumflex branches of left coronary artery, which take blood to back wall of the heart

The aorta (or main artery) conducting blood pumped out of the left pumping chamber (or ventricle) round the body

Left anterior descending coronary artery, which takes blood to front wall of the heart

The right coronary artery

Superior vena cava, which drains blood back from the upper body into the right filling chamber (or atrium)

Apex or 'tip' of the heart

average of 70 times a minute, it will produce somewhere in the region of three billion messages in a 75 year life-span!

Electrical messages from the sinus node spread out through special fibres in the upper chambers to make them beat. These fibres then come together again, rather like tracks converging at a railway junction. Here the messages are held up at another specialised electrical structure close to the right-side inlet valve and this is called the *atrio ventricular node*. The purpose of this node is to delay electrical signals long enough so that the upper chambers (atria) can contract before the lower chambers (ventricles). Once the atria have contracted, the electrical signals pass through the remainder of the heart's wiring system which lies intermingled with the muscle of the ventricles and pass on the messages for the ventricles to contract.

Not only is this wiring system incredibly efficient, but there is also an in-built fail-safe mechanism so that if the main battery fails the atrio ventricular node recognises it has not had any messages from above and can take over and generate messages for the ventricles. Even if both nodes were to fail the ventricles are capable of generating their own electrical impulses, albeit much more slowly than normal, and less reliably. I will turn to this in more detail in Chapter 6.

HEART RATE

The rate at which the heart beats is not constant throughout the day and may change from minute to minute, depending on what we are doing. While we are sleeping, our muscles are at rest, hopefully our minds are too, and the body's need for oxygen is at its lowest. The heart rate may fall as low as 35–40 beats a minute, which in those circumstances is quite acceptable. In the hurly-burly of the rush hour, when you are trying to negotiate a hoard of commuters, all of whom are going in the opposite direction, it is appropriate for the heart rate to go up to 120 or even higher. Under conditions of physical exertion the heart's battery (sinus node) receives messages to instruct it to beat faster. These messages are transmitted both by a special nerve and by a chemical called adrenaline which is produced by a gland near the kidney. After finishing exercise, this mechanism is switched off and the heart gradually slows down. Adrenaline stimulates the heart not only by telling the battery to produce more messages, but also by telling the heart muscle to beat more vigorously. This is why we might notice our hearts pounding after exercise.

A similar mechanism operates under conditions of stress. Sitting in a traffic jam knowing that you are going to be late for the most vital appointment of your life, for example, produces a state of anxiety which mimics the effect of exercise. The heart rate speeds up and the heart seems to pound. It is not only unpleasant experiences like this which increase the heart rate; the same thing also happens when one falls head over heels in love. This mechanism, whereby the heart and circulation adapt to external circumstances, is one of the most basic reactions of animals and is known as the 'flight or fight' reaction, and is central to survival in the jungle or the bush. In the complex animal that is a human being, emotional inputs are just as important as physical ones and, as I will discuss in the chapter on palpitations, anxiety states can often lead people to believe that they have something wrong with their heart.

Certain external influences can also slow the heart abnormally. A classical example of this is the squeamish person who faints at the sight of blood, especially his or her own! A particularly gory scene in a movie can make some people feel sick or dizzy. The heart may slow and, in extreme circumstances, even stop for a few seconds. This reaction is produced by the stimulation of another nerve, called the *vagus nerve*; when the heart slows down, the blood pressure drops and this causes dizziness. The involvement of this nerve has led to the use of the term *vaso vagal attacks* for faints in these circumstances.

I remember a particularly gory scene in a play at The Pit in the Barbican Theatre in London a few years ago. The play, *'Tis Pity She's A Whore* by the post-Shakespearean dramatist John Ford, had as its final scene a banquet with beautiful white linen. Suddenly, and quite unexpectedly, the leading man appears on stage, drenched in blood, holding his lover's heart impaled upon a knife. Blood splashed everywhere. Even as a doctor I felt quite unwell. Looking around me several members of the audience had their heads down between their knees and at least four people were carried out. A more vagal play than this is hard to imagine!

Although the heart is a remarkable machine, it is by no means faultless. Just about every working part of the heart can go wrong, sometimes suddenly and sometimes progressively over time. Most people associate heart disease with arterial blockages and there is no doubt that disease of the coronary arteries is by far the commonest heart disease doctors have to deal with. However, no part of the heart is immune from the disease process. The valves may be attacked by infection and, like any valve, can become blocked or leaky; the electrical circuitry can fail, either through ageing or arterial damage, and the muscle of the heart may become damaged by a variety of factors, including drugs and alcohol.

If you feel fascinated by the workings of this wonderful machine, I hope I can entice you to read on as I do my best to explain the complex topic of heart disease in jargon-free language and how it is likely that people like me will be in business for several years to come.

2

THE ROAD TO CLOGGED-UP ARTERIES

As I explained in Chapter 1, the heart needs a blood supply to function just as any other organ in the body, and the first branches the aorta (the main arterial trunk) gives off turn back on themselves to deliver blood back to the heart muscle. This is rather a strange arrangement, in that the heart needs a good blood supply in order to pump properly, yet it needs to pump properly in order to give itself sufficient blood! It is the only organ in the body which depends upon itself for its nourishment.

The arteries that supply the heart itself, the coronary arteries, can be thought of as motorways which give off A roads which in turn give off B roads until eventually the branches become so small that they cannot be seen with the naked eye or even on x-rays.

There are three coronary arteries, two on the left and one on the right (see diagram, page 22). The right coronary artery is simply called the *right coronary artery*. The artery down the front of the heart on the left is called the *left anterior descending*, which is jargon for 'the artery which runs down the front of the heart on the left' – nothing if not logical! The other left artery is called the *left circumflex*, because it wraps around and towards the back of the heart and often contains quite a few curves.

ARTERIAL DISEASE

These arteries are the fuel pipes of the heart and are

among the most important arteries in the whole body for our survival. Paradoxically, they are also the most vulnerable to furring up and blocking. When we talk about heart disease being the biggest killer in the western world, we nearly always mean disease of these arteries. Deaths due to faulty valves or a faulty electrical system pale into insignificance when compared to the deaths caused by furred-up and blocked coronary arteries. It does seem odd that the arteries upon which we most depend for our lives should also be the most vulnerable to disease. Although other arteries around the body can fur up too, it is common to see people whose arterial tree appears to be in excellent condition except for the coronary arteries in the heart. You might regard this built-in design flaw in these arteries as a way of ensuring we never achieve immortality!

What do I mean by furred-up arteries? What happens is that fatty substances deposit on the wall of the artery and build up over many years. Imagine you are looking down the end of a garden hosepipe. What you would see is a clean circular tube, which is what a normal artery would look like if you could see down it. Now, imagine that someone has put a sticky piece of chewing gum inside the end of the hosepipe. The area through which the water can flow freely is reduced by the gum. If you slowly add more and more chewing gum, the area becomes further reduced. If you block the hosepipe completely with chewing gum, no water will flow out at all. This is exactly what happens to the coronary arteries. The deposition of fatty materials can take decades and we may be totally unaware that it is happening. This process of deposition of fatty material is known as *atherosclerosis* and the deposits themselves are called *atheromatous plaques*. You will hear this furring-up process described in several ways, most commonly as narrowings leading, in

27

cases of severe build-up, to obstructions or blockages.

What happens when the arteries fur up? The diagram on the next page shows points where the atheromatous plaque has obstructed the flow of blood by narrowing the artery. This fatty deposit may take years to develop and many of us are walking around like this without being aware of it.

Furring up or narrowing of the arteries in this way can produce a whole variety of illnesses. Not everyone with deposits in the arteries will develop a heart problem, but the heart cannot function properly if its fuel lines are blocked, in the same way that you would not expect a motor car engine to work if its petrol supply was cut off.

It was through one of the major tragedies of the twentieth century that we learned how early in life fatty deposits on the walls of arteries occur. Many of the young American soldiers who were killed in the Vietnam war were in their late teens or early twenties, and when their bodies were flown home and examined, many of these young men showed evidence of fatty deposition in their arteries. This macabre finding showed that arterial disease begins very early in life. This is of great relevance because if the seeds of furred-up arteries are already sown by the time we reach our late teens then measures to prevent heart disease must be targeted in childhood.

There is an incredibly intimate relationship between the coronary arteries and the heart muscle itself. I often hear patients say: 'His heart was all right, but his arteries were furred up.' If the coronary arteries fur up, or block, either over many years or suddenly, it leads to loss of healthy heart muscle. Although the job of heart specialists is to treat patients' symptoms, we may still recommend treatment when symptoms are not all that severe, in order to prevent the heart muscle being irreversibly damaged, with possibly fatal consequences.

Enlarged portion of the obstructed coronary arteries with a 'window' cut out of the top to show how deposits on the inner wall restrict the area through which blood can flow to the heart muscle

Obstruction in the right coronary artery

Obstructions in the branches of the left coronary artery

RISK FACTORS

So what are the factors that turn the healthy arteries we are born with into the rotten furred-up arteries that may eventually kill us? It has taken years of research to come up with some sensible answers to this question, and even now it is far from fully resolved. The phrase 'There are lies, black lies, and statistics (and, of course, government statistics at the top)' will no doubt be familiar. For example, the rise in coronary deaths in the twentieth century has been paralleled by the rise in ownership of colour televisions and telephones, but it would be ludicrous to infer that heart disease was caused by owning a television or telephone. We need to search for real cause-and-effect relationships rather than assume one thing leads to another, as in the case of heart disease and telephones.

Smoking

Having cautioned against jumping to conclusions, even the most vociferous supporter of the tobacco lobby would have to accept that the link between cigarette smoking and coronary artery diseases is well-established. It is not just being a smoker versus being a non-smoker that counts, but also the degree of smoking. In other words a forty-a-day person has a higher risk of heart disease than a ten-a-day person but the ten-a-day person has a higher risk than a non-smoker. To repeat, heart disease kills far greater numbers than lung cancer does in smokers. Sceptics may quote the anecdotal case of their grandmother who smoked eighty cigarettes a day for sixty years, and lived to be 110, but then this is the exception which proves the rule.

I know that all doctors tell patients to stop smoking, but you only have to wander around a coronary unit for a week or two to see at first hand the devastating effect that cigarette smoking has on people's hearts. The comment: 'But I don't inhale' is rarely greeted by the response of 'Oh well, that's all right, then' by the doctor! The chemicals in the smoke get into the bloodstream and seem to trigger off factors that damage the wall of the artery and promote the deposition of fatty material on the wall. It has recently been shown that smoking low-tar cigarettes is no safer than puffing at the high-tar equivalents in lessening the likelihood of heart attacks. All doctors, and especially those dealing with heart patients, have seen lives and families wrecked by smoking. If I had £5 for every time I heard the words: 'I wish I'd never started smoking, doctor', I would be sailing the Caribbean on a luxury yacht. This is why we are so worried by the rise of cigarette smoking in teenagers, especially in teenage girls (see Chapter 7). Even when people stop smoking, there is evidence that the benefits are gradual and it may take up to twenty years of not smoking before the risk of heart disease is the same as a non-smoker, even though the wallet may benefit immediately!

I quite appreciate that readers might be opposed to a 'nanny state' which tries to tell them what they can eat and what they can inhale into their lungs and might find my observations dogmatic, irritating and offensive. I am also aware of the arguments that smokers pay extra taxes and therefore somehow perceive themselves as paying for their illnesses, but this is, in my view, a rather naive and highly illogical piece of thinking. It is heart specialists like me who are left to pick up the pieces when a heart attack suddenly strikes at a weekend, a bank holiday or on Christmas Day, and consultants are not paid overtime in the NHS. Even if we were, I feel that an attitude of 'I've paid for my heart attack, now get on with making me better' is mentally and physically unhealthy.

If we do not take care of our bodies, we cannot complain

when the doctors charged with the responsibility of putting Humpty Dumpty together again, tell us truths we would rather not hear. After all, if you drive a car that has not been serviced for five years and has never had an oil change or the brake pads renewed, you would not expect praise from the car mechanic who sees how breakdowns and accidents might have been prevented. That said, my sermon on cigarettes will stop here (for the time being!).

Blood pressure

It was only in 1967 that a medical study in America showed that treating blood pressure reduced the death rate. Contrary to popular belief, high blood pressure is not actually a heart disease, although the effects of long-standing high blood pressure can damage the heart in several ways. The muscle of the heart can become thick and high blood pressure is a risk factor for narrowed arteries. It is not only the heart that suffers when blood pressure is high but also other arteries in particular those in the brain, kidneys and eyes.

The situation is complicated by fact that blood pressure tends to rise as we grow older. This means that what we consider normal for someone at 65 or 70 years old may be too high for someone in their thirties. Some difficulty exists in defining what actually is a normal blood pressure, but in one large study in America, a top reading (*systolic*) of 160 millimetres of mercury, or a bottom (*diastolic*) reading of 95 millimetres of mercury, is regarded as abnormal. In this study, patients with elevated blood pressure had twice the incidence of furred-up arteries as people with normal blood pressure.

The life assurance industry carried out a study to predict the reduction in life expectancy caused by raised blood pressure. This was not done for the benefit of patients, but to adjust life assurance premiums in those with high pressure. They calculated that in a 45-year-old woman with a normal blood pressure the life expectancy was 37 years but that it was five years less if the pressure was raised to 145/95 (slightly high) and eight years less if the pressure was 150/100 (moderately high). In men of the same age, the expectancy was 32 years if pressure was normal, and reduced by six years and eleven years for the higher readings.

In populations where coronary heart disease is rife, high blood pressure is one of the most important established risk factors. However, it may produce no symptoms, so people may not be aware that they have high blood pressure and this is obviously dangerous. Treating high blood pressure is one of the best ways of preventing diseased arteries, but it is often difficult to persuade people to take tablets for a condition which produces no symptoms, especially as some of the medicines have side-effects. Patients may perceive their treatment as more of a nuisance than the disease. Furthermore, a doctor receives no pats on the back or Brownie points for the fact that Mr Smith or Mrs Jones did not suffer a heart attack after twenty years of blood pressure-lowering pills!

Cholesterol

It is not just the public that is confused by the information on cholesterol and heart disease. Even in the medical profession, there are evangelists who believe that cholesterol should be abolished from the blood, and those who believe you should eat and drink what you like, and that cholesterol does not matter a hoot. The truth probably lies somewhere between the two extremes. There is now a firm body of scientific evidence that links high cholesterol to the incidence of furred-up coronary arteries – the higher the cholesterol, the greater the risk.

Not only do we take cholesterol in our food, but our bodies manufacture cholesterol. Some people who eat a healthy diet have a high cholesterol level as a result of a defect in the body's metabolism (or chemical factory). Such defects often run in families and at its extreme can cause heart attacks and death even in the twenties and thirties. I know of one tragic case of a 10-year-old dying of a heart attack because of a cholesterol problem. This is not a usual situation, I am glad to say. What is clear, however, is that not all individuals with high cholesterol will fur up their arteries, in the same way that not all smokers will. But, statistically, some well-conducted studies have shown both that high cholesterol contributes to heart disease, and that lowering the cholesterol actually lowers the risk of heart attacks.

The other confusing thing about cholesterol is that there are two main components; a 'good' cholesterol, known as high-density cholesterol, which appears to protect against heart disease, and a 'bad' cholesterol, known as low-density cholesterol, which is responsible for furring up the arteries.

It has been known for about ten years that the rate of furring up of arteries could be slowed down by reducing the levels of low-density cholesterol. However, even in the cholesterol-obsessed USA, treatment did not focus on this. Some of the early cholesterol-lowering research trials used a small number of patients who were followed up for only a short time, and the results showed little impact on the degree of furring up of the arteries. Despite this, the clinical impact of cholesterol lowering was much higher than might have been predicted; in other words, although the arteries remained narrow and furred up, the incidence of heart attacks and the need for heart surgery was reduced.

How could this be? The answer, which still needs to be proved conclusively, is that reducing low-density cholesterol somehow stabilises the arterial narrowings, and reduced the likelihood of these deposits blocking the artery completely. Lowering cholesterol may take the detonator away from the time-bomb. The artery may look to the naked eye like a hosepipe or bony tube, but the arterial wall is very lively and active, beavering away to produce all sorts of chemicals. A high cholesterol level may injure the wall's chemical factory, and lowering it may improve the factory.

There are further subdivisions of cholesterol which are too complex to go into in a book like this, but the bottom line is that heart specialists are becoming more positive in attitude towards lowering cholesterol in people who are perceived as being at high risk, but we *still* do not know whether everybody with a high cholesterol level should be treated. In other words, an isolated high cholesterol count in somebody with no other risk factors and whose living relatives have all received telegrams from the Queen, may not need to be treated the same as somebody with a high cholesterol level who is a smoker and who comes from a family where every member died of heart disease before the age of fifty!

As recently as 1994 surveys in America showed that cholesterol lowering was not uniformly practised in patients with advanced coronary narrowings who had undergone balloon treatment to open up their arteries (this is all explained in Chapter 10). Incredibly, only 22 per cent of males and 25 per cent of females had their cholesterol measured and only half of those with raised cholesterol were treated! Two recently published large research trials have changed our perception of raised cholesterol and we now recognise how important it is to lower cholesterol levels in these patients in order to reduce the incidence of heart attacks.

Diet

Diet is another important risk factor. Many British people have far too much fat in their diet and not enough fibre such as fruit and vegetables. As an unreformable crisp and peanut addict who is not averse to the odd biscuit and who takes sugar in both tea and coffee, I may be accused of hypocrisy by counselling against over-indulgence in these foods. Nevertheless, it would be common sense to reach for the orange pieces at a party instead of the crisp bowl. The debate over margarine and butter goes beyond whether one can tell the difference between them, but whether or not it really matters. Compared with smoking, eating foods from these categories does not matter very much. However, a balanced diet of fresh food and a reduction in the intake of processed food would appear sensible.

One of the most confusing things for the public is the continued use of jargon terms, such as 'polyunsaturated' and 'saturated' fatty acids. These terms refer to the chemical structure of certain fatty materials which exist in meat, fish and dairy products. It has generally been held that saturated fatty acids are bad for you, and raise your cholesterol level, whereas polyunsaturated fatty acids are good for you and lower your cholesterol level. Unfortunately it is not so simple, and researchers are currently trying to unravel the various mysteries of the different forms of acids. Some acids appear to be more likely to produce furred-up arteries than others. Milk, butter and cheese in a diet tend to make one more prone to produce furred-up arteries by increasing the levels of the low-density cholesterol, whereas some seed and fish oil may protect against blood clots.

If we accept that dietary habits may influence the development of arterial disease at an early age, and that arterial disease is the penalty we pay for having enough, or rather too much to eat and not dying of infectious diseases, famine, drought or civil war, then the least we can do is to educate our children in proper eating habits, as well as discourage them from smoking. I recently stayed in a wonderful hotel in America (the fear of legal action precludes me from telling you which one!) where one of its many restaurants had two menus. The adult menu detailed exactly how many high- and low-density ingredients each dish contained and announced proudly that the menu had been approved by the American Heart Association. It included such worthy ingredients as fresh fish, pasta and olive oil, and was, indeed, impressive. The children's menu contained the following:

CHILDREN'S MENU
Pizza with nut and jam topping
Mega-burger of prime beef with double cheese topping
Big Fat Wizard Waffles with loads of whipped cream and extra syrup
Chocolate pudding with chocolate cake and choice of chocolate and syrup sauce with biscuits and extra cream.

You may well ask what sort of demonic caterer had dreamed up a menu, which would have the local dentists rubbing their hands with glee at the thought of the lucrative work being so carefully prepared for them, and at the same time sow the seeds for the next generation of heart disease statistics. The irony is that, given the location of the hotel, the Heart Association-approved menu was being fed to people of whom a large proportion had already had at least one, maybe two (even three!) coronary by-pass operations, so that it was too late to matter. But to a generation of clean arterial specimens, they were quite prepared to feed the menu from Hell! When I telephoned the vice-president in charge of catering, and pointed out what he was doing to the children, he replied: 'This is a corporate menu, sir.' I am not quite sure what I was supposed to say to that, but what I did say is unprintable!

Obesity

The public's image of someone likely to be at risk from a heart attack is of a grossly overweight person and certainly many doctors have this attitude as well. Scientifically, however, being 'horizontally' or 'circumferentially' challenged, may not actually be a risk factor for narrowed or blocked arteries. This is because there are so many other things that tend to go with being obese, such as high blood pressure, a high cholesterol level and physical inactivity. The pendulum has thus swung the other way, with many bright sparks making statements that being overweight or obese doesn't actually matter. Stop! Before you reach for the refrigerator door or another bag of crisps, do understand that being overweight probably does contribute to an increased likelihood of having other risk factors which cause heart attacks. Weight loss will have beneficial effects on cholesterol and blood pressure, as well as general physical well-being. Remember that obesity does not just contribute to deadly heart attacks, but can also lead to other less serious but equally disabling conditions, such as arthritis, in later life.

Age and sex

In both sexes the death rate from furred-up arteries increases with age. It is probable that age in its own right has only a minor effect on the incidence of furred-up and blocked arteries, and that it is the cumulative effect of smoking, high blood pressure and raised cholesterol over time which is more important. Remember, not everybody who has furred-up arteries will have a clinical illness associated with it, and some people die at an advanced age *with* furred-up arteries rather than *of* them.

As far as gender is concerned, there is a big difference in the death rate between men and women, with men between 35 and 44 years old having about a six times greater chance of dying than women of the same age. But as we grow older, that difference diminishes. (The problem of furred-up arteries in women is one that has, until recently, been slightly neglected; and I cover this topic in some detail in Chapter 7.)

Race

Certain ethnic groups have a higher incidence of coronary disease than others. In many cases, this may be due to specific genetic disorders which affect, in particular, blood cholesterol. There is a condition known as *familial hyperlipidaemia*, which means 'high fat levels that run in families'. One often sees advanced arterial narrowings in patients from the Asian subcontinent at a particularly young age, and again, within this group, particularly in women. In contrast, Afro-Caribbeans have a much lower incidence of furred-up arteries even if they have a higher incidence of higher blood pressure. As yet there is no satisfactory explanation for this.

Diabetes

Diabetics have a higher incidence of heart problems than non-diabetics. There is some debate as to whether this is to do with the diabetes or associated conditions often found in diabetics, such as being overweight or having a high cholesterol level or high blood pressure. Again, diabetes seems to carry a higher risk in women.

Family history

It is now generally accepted that a bad family medical history (defined as clinical evidence of furred-up arteries before the age of 50 in a first-degree relative, such as a brother or sister or parent), constitutes an important risk factor. Sometimes other risk factors such as high blood pressure, diabetes and high cholesterol run in families, making it hard to determine whether family history has an independent effect transmitted through generation to generation. I am occasionally asked to see someone who has had no symptoms, but who has had four or five brothers die before the age of 50. If it turns out that all these brothers were heavy smokers and the man I am seeing is not, does that mean that this individual will develop heart disease? Of course, nobody knows. It does seem likely that there is some susceptibility for developing arterial disease which is transmitted from generation to generation, and this may interact with other factors such as smoking and blood pressure which will cause the problem. We often say, jokingly, that people should choose their parents correctly, but many a true word is spoken in jest!

Physical activity

It is hard to define the role of exercise or lack of it and its relationship to furring-up arteries or heart attacks. Being physically active tends to reduce weight and keep one mobile, and there is also evidence to suggest that a heart attack is less likely to be fatal in exercisers than in non-exercisers. But it is difficult to identify the true role of exercise here, because people who pursue fitness are likely to be more conscious about keeping their weight down, of not smoking, having their blood pressure checked more regularly and eating a healthy diet. Physical inactivity can be a major problem among women, who tend to be less active than their male counterparts.

Personality and stress

This is a difficult area to study scientifically. In the 1950s, two personality traits, known as Type A and Type B, were identified. The Type A person (interestingly enough, a man not a woman!) was classified as an aggressive, over-ambitious, time-conscious, over-competitive, impatient, abrupt individual, who is constantly chasing his tail and engaged in 'a chronic and obsessive struggle, to obtain an unlimited number of things from the environment'! Many of us are Type A individuals to a greater or lesser degree.

The Type B individual is the laid-back, chilled-out, relaxed, unambitious person whose life goes along at its own steady pace, regardless of how others expect him or her to work.

Some early research suggested that Type A behaviour was an independent risk factor for heart attacks and many of us would view such individuals who race around in permanent competition with themselves and everybody else as heading for heart attacks. The problem with making such an assumption is that Type A individuals are also more likely to be heavy smokers, take little exercise and run high levels of blood pressure.

The Type A individual may thrive on adrenaline, but is it actually a good thing? The axiom that hard work never killed anyone may be medically correct, but there does come a time in life when deadlines, demanding bosses and a 16-hour working day take their toll, even if there is a Porsche in the garage as some consolation. I recognise the SOBB (Stressed Out Beyond Belief) syndrome among my colleagues and my patients and, I hate to say, even in myself. Bereavement, difficulties at work, problems with a

41

spouse or partner can all affect the heart as well as one's sense of well-being. These sorts of stresses raise the level of the chemical adrenaline in the blood which causes the heart to beat faster and blood pressure to rise. Surges in blood pressure may contribute to blood clots forming on narrowed segments of arteries. Adrenaline may also cause other chemicals (called free fatty acids) to rise in the blood and these can sometimes be a stimulus for changes in the heart's rhythm.

I remember one patient, normally a calm, placid individual, who was stuck in a traffic jam on the motorway and started to worry about an important appointment. He passed from the sighing to the foot-tapping stage, but still the traffic did not move. Next came the beads of sweat on the brow and that awful, sticky feeling around the collar which progressed rapidly to the ape-like bashing of his hands against the steering wheel. When his temper could not be contained within the vehicle, he got out of his car and paced up and down the line of stationary traffic and began to hurl abuse at the other drivers in front of him. What he had not bargained for was the reaction of a similarly frustrated driver, an ex-army, amateur boxing champion, who proceeded to execute a perfect right hook on my patient's jaw!

As my patient recalled at a later date, it was only when the fierce pain in his face was replaced by a worse one in his chest that he realised that something might be amiss. Needless to say, he did not make the appointment and ended up in the local coronary unit with a heart attack. As he had no other identifiable risk factors for his illness, he took some convincing when I tried to point out that although stress was not likely to be a primary cause of heart disease, excessive stress was important in producing the first clinical sign of heart disease in arteries that were already abnormal. In other words, the incident was there waiting to happen because his arteries were already slightly furred up. Clearly, if he had not found himself in the circumstances in which he did, the illness would probably not have surfaced at that time.

Apart from work, some other stresses in my own life, with which some of you may have some sympathy, are:

- Receiving a tax demand from the Inland Revenue.
- Receiving a telephone bill with a teenage daughter in the house.
- Supporting Chelsea Football Club.

Any Chelsea fans reading this book will surely recognise this, as the club has over the past three decades put its supporters through the pain barrier. My passionate devotion to the club prevents me from turning my allegiance elsewhere, but at what cost to my coronary arteries? Still, at least at Chelsea you go down fighting with a heart attack, whereas Arsenal fans just die of boredom!

To sum up, as far as stress is concerned, if your arteries are healthy you are unlikely to come to any harm, but stress may well bring things to a head if your arteries are already furred up. The screen image of a man clutching his chest when confronted by bad news is not all that far from the truth.

Although we have managed to identify many risk factors associated with clogged-up arteries, the true cause remains something of a mystery. Many people have artery problems who on the face of it do not deserve them, so life is unfair, even when it comes to heart disease.

3

THE ACHING HEART AND HEART ATTACKS

What sort of illnesses can narrowed or blocked coronary arteries produce? The diseases caused by arterial problems are known as *ischaemic* (pronounced is-kee-mick) heart disease, meaning heart short of oxygen. When the heart is short of blood, for example, it is called *myocardial ischaemia*. These diseases include pain from the heart muscle, heart attacks, sudden death and heart failure. I will explain what each of these are and why they occur, why it may be difficult for doctors to get a good feel for patients' symptoms, and also why doctors may fail to ask the right questions.

HEART PAIN (ANGINA)

The heart's job is to pump blood around the body. The bulk of the heart is muscle and any muscle needs a blood supply. As long as supply equals demand everything is rosy, and in normal circumstances the arteries are capable of delivering enough blood to the heart. However, the needs of the heart will differ in varying circumstances. While we are asleep it is not asked to do much work and needs a relatively small amount of blood. But if we are running up several flights of stairs or playing tennis (or watching Chelsea!), it needs more oxygen because it is being asked to pump faster to deliver more blood around the body. The coronary arteries are therefore asked to supply more blood into the heart muscle.

If the arteries are normal or only minimally narrowed, the coronary arteries can deliver as much oxygen as the heart needs. But if the arteries become obstructed (as shown in the diagram on page 29) they will only be capable of supplying the demands of the heart at rest. When playing tennis, running for a bus or up the stairs, demand will exceed supply and the heart becomes short of oxygen. At this stage the heart muscle may hurt. This is known as *angina*. Angina is not a disease, but a symptom, in the same way that toothache or headache is a symptom.

To understand this concept of muscles hurting, raise your left arm above your head and clench and unclench your fist as fast as you can. You are making the muscles of your forearm work hard so that they require more oxygen, while limiting the blood supply by making the heart pump against gravity. After a while your forearm – and possibly your hand – will begin to hurt. This pain is caused by the build-up of chemicals produced by muscles and these chemicals are not cleared quickly enough by the blood. As soon as you stop exercising your arm and lower it to your side the pain will subside. This is exactly what happens when the heart muscle hurts. Angina is cramp from the heart muscle – it is heartache in the truest sense.

People's experiences vary and many patients do not perceive these feelings as a true pain and find it hard to describe the symptoms. The word 'angina' comes from the Latin word meaning strangulation. The classic description of angina is a heavy, strangling, vice-like or tight feeling in the chest.

Some people believe that pain from the heart must be located where the heart is, i.e. over the left side of the chest. They think that if pain is on the right side it cannot be from the heart. Other people feel that if the pain does not go into their arms or their throat, it cannot be heart pain, while yet others believe that if the pain goes down the right arm but not the left it cannot be heart pain. None of these is true.

The sensation of tightness, pain or ache can be felt in the centre, right or left-hand side of the chest, may or may not go down the arms or into the throat, or may be felt only in the arm. Occasionally, pain from the heart can radiate up into the jaw, chin or teeth, and into the wrists or fingers.

The doctors have read the text books but our hearts have not, so not all angina pain will go down the left arm or into the jaw or make the patient short of breath or sweaty. Most heart specialists will have seen patients with only jaw pain or even toothache, or pain only felt in their thumb or inner arm. I had a patient referred to me from a dentist, who made the diagnosis of angina when his patient said that he only felt toothache when hurrying for a train in the morning. The reason that pain from the heart often goes down the arm or into the jaw relates to the heart's nerve supply. Pain felt in locations other than the chest is known as *referred pain*.

The skilled doctor will tease out of a patient a good description of the symptoms, although sometimes this requires the patience of Job and the persistence of Lieutenant Columbo! Such a doctor will also look for evidence which would support a diagnosis of heart pain, such as accompanying shortness of breath or sweating. Observations by relatives and friends who notice a change in skin colour to a grey, sweaty appearance may be important.

Before any doctor can exercise any form of skill, however, the patient has to seek medical advice – no one teaches us telepathy at medical school! It is amazing how many people attribute their symptoms of chest discomfort to that dreaded word 'indigestion'. If I had my way I would strike it from the English language. At least 7 out of 10 patients I see, who end up with a diagnosis of angina, have assumed they are suffering from indigestion. To put it bluntly, the mortuaries are full of people with 'indigestion'.

I remember while attending cardiac arrest calls in casualty at Bart's (before the government closed our department down) that there would often be the dreaded bottle of chalky white medicine in the victim's pocket. If only one reader realises that he or she should consult a doctor as a result of what I have written, I will have achieved something.

Indigestion is usually felt in the abdomen, not in the chest or behind the breast bone. It should have no relationship to physical activity. Even doctors misdiagnose their own symptoms! I have doctors as patients who have ignored their own typical heart pain, attributing it to a peanut overdose or a bout of flu, whereas if the same symptoms had been given to them by one of their patients they would have called an ambulance.

However, heart pain can be associated with a desire to bring up wind, and people often assume that if they do this they have indigestion or over-acidity. Another confusing aspect is that angina can occur when walking after a meal, and some patients may only exhibit symptoms if they exert themselves after a meal. The body diverts blood to the digestive system after eating, and to the limb muscles during physical activity. If the arteries are narrowed the heart cannot cope simultaneously with the demands of digestion and exercise – hence the pain.

Heart pain which occurs with exertion is known as *angina of effort*. People may not perceive ordinary physical activity as effort, but even a hundred-metre walk on level ground or a smaller distance up a slope makes the heart do more work than it has to do at rest and may provoke symptoms. Heart specialists can predict an increase in the number of people referred with angina at certain times of the year, for example when mowing the grass for the first time in spring, shovelling snow in winter, or walking in the first cold or windy morning of the year.

Patients may not necessarily get angina every time they undertake a certain level of exertion. Some days, for example, they might be able to walk a few miles without any discomfort but on another day they might find that the pain begins after only after a few strides. This is because it is possible for the heart to be short of blood yet not produce any symptoms. The fact that you may not get pain every time you walk should not therefore put you off visiting your doctor.

Another term for chest pain on exertion is *stable angina*. This is very common and many people can live with stable angina for a long time. The seriousness of angina relates not to the unpleasant feeling it may cause, but to its implications, i.e. whether the symptoms represent a potentially life-threatening condition or not. The severity of the chest pain or discomfort bears little relation to the seriousness of the problem, so it is possible to have mild angina and yet have a life-threatening disease or, conversely, to have bad angina which is not caused by life-threatening narrowings. Stable angina may or may not worsen over time.

Unstable angina is a completely different symptom. It can occur in one of two ways. First, a patient with stable angina may experience a sudden change in symptoms, where attacks become more frequent, more severe and last longer, and may be less responsive to medication. Pain may also occur for the first time on minimal exertion (such as walking from one room to another) or even at rest. It may also wake people up in the middle of the night. Secondly, unstable angina may occur in somebody who has never had any symptoms before. Chest pain at rest or at night should start alarm bells ringing.

If someone has become used to having angina when they overdo things, they may recognise that something is amiss when they experience symptoms in unusual circumstances, but even 'experienced' heart patients often fail to recognise symptoms as coming from the heart, simply because they do not understand that they can have heart pain at rest. In somebody who has never experienced heart pain, sudden discomfort in the chest may not be attributed to the heart, but due, I am afraid, to indigestion! However, unstable angina is a medical emergency and if not treated properly can lead to a full-blown heart attack.

Nobody who goes to a casualty department with symptoms of chest discomfort at rest or on minimal exertion should be sent home. They should be admitted to hospital immediately and placed on a drip. Even if you are faced with an inexperienced doctor in casualty (as can happen!) you can help yourself by knowing what symptoms to look for and insisting the doctor take them seriously. The long waits in casualty departments give ample opportunity for the symptoms to subside.

Take the following example of a doctor/patient interview in casualty.

CASUALTY OFFICER:	Sorry to keep you. It has been very busy in here. What seems to be the problem?
PATIENT:	Well, I feel fine now, but I had this strange feeling in my chest.
CASUALTY OFFICER:	When was this?
PATIENT:	About four hours ago. I was just climbing into bed when it started.
CASUALTY OFFICER:	Can you show me where you felt the pain?
PATIENT:	Yes, it was here, across my chest. Just like indigestion.
CASUALTY OFFICER:	Was it like a burning sensation? Did it go anywhere else?

PATIENT: It was hard to describe. It wasn't really burning and I didn't feel it anywhere else.

CASUALTY OFFICER: And it has all gone, now, has it?

PATIENT: Yes, I feel fine now.

The casualty officer briefly examines the patient.

CASUALTY OFFICER: Well, I can't find anything. We will just get an ECG [this is short for Electrocardiogram and is a print-out of the heartbeat] and a chest x-ray done. I am afraid there will be a bit of a wait.

PATIENT: Have I had a heart attack, doctor?

CASUALTY OFFICER: I think that's very unlikely, but we will just do an ECG and chest x-ray to be on the safe side.

An ECG and chest x-ray will then be carried out.

CASUALTY OFFICER: You'll be glad to know there is nothing on your cardiogram or x-ray, so I think you will be all right. Please take this note to your GP and he may ask you to see a heart specialist.

PATIENT: Thank you, doctor. Can I go home, now?

CASUALTY OFFICER: Yes, I think so.

This whole process may have taken some hours. Unlike a television series, there may not be a consultant or highly experienced doctor around 24 hours a day. Many hospitals, but not all, have a policy that patients with chest pain must be seen by the on-call medical registrar, who may be more experienced. Even then, patients whose chest pains have disappeared and whose ECGs are normal are often discharged from hospital instead of being kept in under observation. Cases have occurred where patients who have been discharged have then suffered a full-blown heart attack, or even died suddenly, a short time later.

If someone is having such a heart attack, changes do occur on the ECG. However – just to complicate things – the ECG may be normal in unstable angina even during the attack or once the pain has gone. So, although the ECG is useful if it shows changes, the fact that it does not show changes may lull doctors into a false sense of security. The patient's medical history is much more important than a wiggly line on a piece of paper (which is what the ECG is). Here is how the interview should have taken place:

CASUALTY OFFICER: Sorry to keep you. It has been very busy in here. What seems to be the problem?

PATIENT: Well, I feel fine now, but I had this strange feeling in my chest.

CASUALTY OFFICER: When was this?

PATIENT: About four hours ago. I was just climbing into bed when it started.

CASUALTY OFFICER: Can you show me where you felt the pain?

PATIENT: Yes, it was here, across my chest. Just like indigestion.

CASUALTY OFFICER: Was it like a burning sensation? Did it go anywhere else?

PATIENT:	Well, it was hard to describe. It wasn't really burning and I didn't feel it anywhere else.
CASUALTY OFFICER:	And it has all gone, now, has it?
PATIENT:	Yes, I feel fine now.
CASUALTY OFFICER:	How long do you think this sensation lasted, altogether.
PATIENT:	About twenty minutes or so.
CASUALTY OFFICER:	If it wasn't a burning sensation, can you try and describe it for me using some other terms.
PATIENT:	Well, as I say, it was like indigestion; but quite severe.
CASUALTY OFFICER:	Was it a heavy or tight sort of feeling.
PATIENT:	Yes, I suppose it was tightness more than pain.
CASUALTY OFFICER:	Are you a smoker? Or do you have high blood pressure or diabetes?
PATIENT:	I haven't smoked for five years. I haven't had my blood pressure taken for ages.
CASUALTY OFFICER:	Has anyone in your family had heart trouble?
PATIENT:	Well, my father had some sort of heart thrombosis and my older brother had a heart by-pass operation.

The casualty officer examines the patient. By asking a few

more relevant questions the doctor has established that the feeling in the chest was a tightness, that the patient is an ex-smoker and has a family history of heart disease. The ECG and x-ray will now be carried out, after which the interview continues:

CASUALTY OFFICER: Well, it seems unlikely there is any damage to the heart. But we have to be suspicious that the pain is coming from the heart. The right thing to do is to keep you in hospital, if only for a couple of days.

PATIENT: Is that really necessary, doctor?

CASUALTY OFFICER: I am afraid so. We can't rule out the possibility of an impending heart attack and it would be much safer for you to be in hospital, rather than roaming around the streets. We need to run some blood tests, start you on aspirin to thin the blood and probably try some other medications as well.

Not every patient who comes to casualty with chest pain that has subsequently subsided has unstable angina. Pain that is felt as a pricking sensation that lasts only a few seconds very rarely originates from the heart, but it is important to exclude the most serious possibility, namely unstable angina. If that proves not to be the case, the doctor can go on to investigate other organs, such as the stomach.

The medical history is of paramount importance. There is wide variation in the standard of patient histories taken by GPs, and some GPs will refer any patient with a symptom between the neck and the belly button to casualty or to outpatients with a possible diagnosis of heart pain. There is a wonderful (true!) story of a GP who was notoriously idle. One night, a patient knocked on his door and received no answer. The patient persisted and after several minutes an upstairs window opened, and the doctor leaned out:

DOCTOR: What's the matter, then?

PATIENT: I've got a chest pain, doctor.

DOCTOR: Just a minute.

The patient expected to be let in and examined, but instead a piece of paper floated down from the upstairs window and landed at the patient's feet. It was the top of a cereal packet! 'Take this to casualty,' cried the doctor. The patient did as he was told. Upon arrival he handed in his 'referral letter', which read:

> Dear Doctor,
> Query heart?
> Yours faithfully, etc.

The patient was quite properly seen and examined, and given a note to take back to his GP. The note from casualty read:

> Dear Doctor,
> Heart present.
> Yours faithfully,
> Casualty Officer

I digress. Why should angina that has been stable suddenly become unstable? Why should symptoms arise out of the blue, in someone who has had no symptoms before? Referring back to the demand/supply equation, if angina pain occurs at rest it implies that supply has decreased even though demand remains the same. We know that the deposits that fur up the arteries become larger with time and that, at a certain point, the obstruction to blood flow down the artery may become so great that flow is reduced even at rest.

Coronary arteries are living tissue and around the inner lining of the artery is a muscular 'coat', which is capable of contracting and relaxing. If the muscular coat goes into spasm, it reduces the area through which blood can flow. The purpose of some of the tablets used to treat unstable angina is to relax the muscular coat of the artery. Another, and probably the most important, reason is that a small blood clot develops suddenly, narrowing the artery even further and reducing the supply of blood.

Treatment for this condition includes bed rest, the administration of a drug called heparin through a drip, and aspirin tablets. These drugs thin the blood and stop new blood clots forming. Nearly all patients with unstable angina will stabilise on medical treatment and should have the necessary tests later.

Although unstable angina is a serious condition, if treated properly the patient may escape without damage to the heart muscle. However, if not treated properly, the condition may progress to a full-blown heart attack. Unstable angina may be regarded as a 'pre-shock' or warning of a heart attack to follow, just as a major earthquake is preceded by tremors.

HEART ATTACK

The term *heart attack* is misleading because theoretically any attack of chest pain that comes from the heart should be regarded as a heart attack. In practice, however, the term is reserved for a specific illness where part of the heart muscle is killed by a total, or near total, obstruction in the artery, preventing blood flowing down the artery on which the muscle depends. The technical description is a *myocardial infarction* (meaning 'death of the heart muscle'). The word 'infarction' comes from the Latin, meaning 'to stuff' – when you look at the heart under a microscope, it becomes stuffed full of cells to help heal the damage. Another term you will hear to describe a heart attack is *coronary thrombosis* (often shortened to *coronary*) which means a blood clot in a coronary artery.

Remember that although nobody dies from angina people do die of heart attacks. Statistics show that there are 22 deaths an hour in Britain from heart attacks. So what actually happens and why?

We can answer the first part of the question but not the second. The fatty deposit on the arterial wall, shown in the diagram on page 29, has a covering of fibrous tissue (or cap). This tissue can be thought of as a thin layer of skin-like material. It may remain stable as the fatty material grows over decades; indeed, many of us have such deposits or plaques which will never bother us. However, the tissue sometimes ruptures like the top blowing off a volcano and this can occur as unpredictably as a volcanic eruption. What causes this 'time bomb' to detonate we do not fully understand, but – as we saw in Chapter 2 – cholesterol may be a factor, as may surges in blood pressure.

When this happens, blood flowing through the artery comes into contact with the fatty deposits and a blood clot forms, mushrooming from the fatty tissue and obstructing the artery. Supply is totally cut off and the heart muscle, suddenly deprived of blood, screams out in agony. As with angina, the pain can run up into the jaw or down the arms and is often accompanied by shortness of breath and profuse sweating. Symptoms may last for several hours. The clinical picture may vary from the full-blown symptoms just described to a milder feeling of discomfort which people often ignore. Cutting off the blood supply to the heart muscle, like any other muscle, will kill it.

Some people will die before they have had time to complain of chest pain. The reason this happens is that when the heart muscle is suddenly deprived of blood, it may become electrically unstable, which means that instead of beating, the pumping chambers (ventricles) first shiver or vibrate in a chaotic way. Rhythm disturbances can be seen on an ECG and the most common is called *ventricular fibrillation (VF)*. When the heart stops pumping, this is called a *cardiac arrest*. Blood flow to all other organs, including the brain, then ceases and the patient rapidly loses consciousness. Hopefully, many of you will have done resuscitation courses which show you how to preserve blood flow to the brain by performing cardiac massage and by making sure that enough oxygen gets into the bloodstream by giving mouth-to-mouth resuscitation. When the public sees sense, and I am finally declared dictator, one of the first laws I will pass is to make it essential for people to do life support courses. When the ambulance arrives or when the patient reaches casualty an electric shock will be administered, using a machine called a *defibrillator*, which restarts the heart. You may have seen this in television dramas.

Sudden, unheralded death can be the first and only symptom in between a fifth and a quarter of all heart attacks and appears to be more common in young and middle-aged adults than in the older population. Of all people who die of heart attacks, between 40 and 60 per cent will die before they arrive in hospital. The problem for doctors is how to identify something so unpredictable as the rupture of the plaque and the formation of a blood clot, which can occur in people who appear to be extremely healthy. It is even possible for someone to have undergone a full medical screen, including a walking test on a treadmill, and to die the next day. Paradoxically, it is the less severe deposits that rupture suddenly, minor obstructions being difficult to detect. Statistically, if a patient makes it to hospital, he or she is already past the most dangerous period. If serious rhythm disturbances arise in hospital they can be promptly dealt with, either in casualty or in the coronary care unit.

Clot-buster drugs

One of the medical revolutions of the last decade has been the arrival of the 'clot-buster' drugs. These are given to restore flow through the blocked artery and to reduce or prevent damage to the heart muscle. They are injected directly through a vein while powerful drugs like heroin are given for pain relief and oxygen is given through a mask.

Clot-buster drugs must be given as quickly as possible, because one of the major factors in dictating how well a patient will recover depends upon how much heart muscle has been killed by losing its blood supply. When doctors talk about 'mild', 'severe' or even 'massive' (how I hate this word!) heart attacks, they are referring, not to the severity of the patients' symptoms, but to how much damage has been done. Prompt delivery of clot-busting drugs and restoration of blood flow can change what was destined to be a severe heart attack into a less severe or mild attack. In some cases, they can prevent any damage being done at all. That does not mean that the symptoms of a mild heart attack are any less horrible than those of a big one. We would no doubt be just as terrified in an earthquake that measured 4 or 5 on the Richter Scale as in an earthquake measuring 8.

The way you can help is by not sitting on your symptoms. There is little we can do to save precious heart muscle if you do not seek medical advice. So when that heavy, crushing, vice-like chest pain or tightness comes on, get thee to a hospital pretty damned quick!

Many casualty departments have a system called *triaging* on arrival, so that patients who look as though they are having a heart attack are treated immediately and given the clot-busting drugs as quickly as possible. Mistakes will sometimes be made as some people who should have the drug will not be given it, and some people who do not need it, will be. Because these drugs dissolve blood clots, they can also make the patient bleed and someone with a bleeding stomach ulcer, or who has recently undergone a major operation or suffered from a brain haemorrhage, for example, will not be a suitable candidate. There is a quick checklist that doctors should follow before deciding if it is safe to proceed with this kind of treatment.

After clot-busting drugs have been given, most patients will be given aspirin. This is not given for pain relief but because it makes certain cells in the blood less sticky and less likely to form blood clots.

Electrocardiograms (ECGs)

The next question is how to tell when someone is simply having an attack of unstable angina or suffering a full-blown heart attack. Apart from the patient's medical history, which includes the duration of the pain, the diagnosis is established by doing an ECG. For people who have not had an ECG before, the process of being wired up around the hands, feet and chest and seeing the wiggly lines being produced on paper can be quite frightening. The machine is not putting electricity through the heart, but merely translating the heartbeat into an electrical signal which can be read. Sometimes, simultaneously, the heartbeat comes up on a monitor, accompanied by that familiar beeping noise.

The ECG will show signs of damage to the heart muscle. In order to avoid giving the clot-busting drugs inappropriately, doctors set certain criteria on the ECG before the drugs are administered. Before you remind me that, a few pages back, I said that you could have heart pain and have a normal ECG, remember that I am now referring to a situation where the heart is actually being damaged. Therein lies the difference between unstable angina and a true heart attack. In the former, the heart hurts but has not been damaged whereas for a heart attack to have taken place there must be evidence of damage. This may be confusing for patients who hear something like this:

DOCTOR: Well, Mr Burnside, all our tests show that you did not have a heart attack, because all the blood tests and cardiograms have remained normal. But what you did have was a bout of unstable angina or pain coming from the heart. You are better now, so you can go home on these tablets and you will come back for a treadmill test in a few weeks.

You can imagine Mr Burnside trying to come to terms with the apparently conflicting information that he did not have a heart attack but that the pain *had* come from his heart. What the doctor meant to say was that Mr Burnside had suffered from a severe attack of cramp from his heart muscle and he was lucky that there was no damage done. He suffered heart pain, but it was not a heart attack in the true medical sense because a heart attack equals damaged muscle!

Although it is usually obvious from the ECG whether damage has taken place, a heart specialist may seek confirmation of injury to the heart by measuring chemicals in the blood which are released when the muscle is damaged. These chemicals are known as *cardiac enzymes*. In healthy heart muscle they are contained within the cells and only a small amount is measurable in the bloodstream. When the heart muscle is damaged the cells release these enzymes into the blood. Levels go up in the first few days, before gradually falling to normal.

Patients will also usually have a chest x-ray carried out to assess the size of the heart and to see if the lungs are congested. In mild heart attacks there may be no noticeable effects on the circulation because there is enough healthy heart muscle left to take over. The greater the muscle damage, the more likelihood there is that the pumping function of the heart will become defective.

AFTERCARE

Most people make a good recovery from a heart attack, but nationwide the level of aftercare is something of a lottery. Some parts of the UK are well served by heart units and well-trained heart specialists. Other areas are not so lucky. In some cases (particularly when patients do not have access to a heart specialist) patients may be seen once or twice in outpatients and then simply told to get on with their lives. Often this happens when heart attack victims are not looked after by heart specialists but by physicians who specialise in other areas, such as stomach problems, diabetes or kidney disease. General physicians are perfectly capable of looking after heart attack patients in the early stages but it is what happens afterwards which is so variable.

If a heart attack is uncomplicated, patients are usually off work for a couple of months. Strict attention should be paid to risk factors, which include giving up smoking, controlling blood pressure, checking cholesterol level (if necessary, being given drugs to lower it) and losing weight. Of these, giving up smoking and losing weight are the most difficult, though I generally find there is nothing so good at making people stop smoking as having the living daylights scared out of them.

Many patients will be placed on medication, most commonly drugs known as beta-blockers. Research carried out some years ago showed that death and recurrent heart attack rates were reduced when patients were placed on these drugs. However, some people are not destined to have another attack, even if they do not take beta-blockers, and some people will have another heart attack in spite of taking the drugs. This 'blanket therapy' is fine if no other tests are planned but it makes no sense to whack everybody onto a beta-blocker and hope for the best if we have tests available that help decide if patients are at a low, medium or high risk for having future attacks. Chapter 10 deals with the treatments available.

COMPLICATIONS

Not all heart attacks run an uncomplicated course. Although the clot-busting drugs have reduced death rates, it is still advisable for patients to go to coronary care units so that the heart rhythm can be monitored for the first days after an attack.

Further blood clots

Other complications in the early stages include the formation of another blood clot at the same site in the artery, which will usually produce more chest pain and be accompanied by new changes on the ECG. It may be necessary to give a second dose of clot-buster drug and where the clot keeps re-forming the patient may need to be transferred urgently to a hospital which has all the equipment for x-raying inside the heart in order to deal with the problem. Treatment will involve either balloon technology or heart surgery (see Chapter 10).

Occasionally a blood clot forms *inside* the cavity of the damaged pumping chamber (ventricle) and this type of clot can break off, move out of the heart and get stuck elsewhere in the circulation. A clot that starts in one place and moves to another is called an *embolism*. If the clot ends up in the brain it may cause a stroke. These clots are usually associated with heart attacks involving the front wall of the heart and doctors will often do an ultrasonic examination of the heart in such patients, as clots like these may show up on such scans. If a clot is present the patient will need to go onto blood-thinning medication for a few months, or even permanently.

Ruptures

Other mechanical problems can develop which might require immediate transfer to a heart unit. If the heart attack damages the attachments of the left inlet valve, the valve can rupture and leak torrentially backwards towards the lungs. Similarly, the septum or heart's 'wall', dividing the left side of the heart from the right, may rupture, allowing blood to flow from the left pumping chamber to the right pumping chamber. This is called a *ventricular septal defect*.

Both a leaking valve and a septal defect usually make a patient very ill, because the heart is put under an enormous strain. Treatment is geared towards making the patient fit to undergo either a repair or replacement of the leaking valve, or repair of the septal defect. Even with this complex and intensive treatment, rupture of the left inlet valve or a ventricular septal defect caused by a heart attack are grave conditions and even in the most expert hands people may not survive, despite early surgery.

A greater catastrophe can occur if the damaged heart muscle ruptures and blood leaks out into the lining of the heart. This 'bleeding heart' is invariably fatal, but fortunately uncommon.

Inflamed heart lining

Sometimes the lining of the heart becomes inflamed after a heart attack. This can cause a pain similar to the original one, but is more likely to be made worse by breathing in, changing body position or coughing. This is called *pericarditis* and can be calmed down by some simple anti-inflammatory medication. It rarely produces long-term complications.

The shocked heart

Most of the serious complications relate to the degree of damage to the heart muscle. The more muscle is damaged the worse the condition becomes. In extreme circumstances, the brain may not get enough blood and the patient becomes confused; the kidneys do not get enough blood so the amount of urine produced decreases, and the blood vessels in the skin constrict, which may make the patient cold and sweaty. This condition is called *cardiogenic shock* (cardiogenic means 'caused by the heart', and shock (which does not mean 'fright' here) refers to a specific illness characterised by low blood pressure, confusion and reduced urine output. This can be fatal. The incidence of this appears to have decreased since the appearance of clot-

busting drugs, but it still occurs now and then and the outlook is grave.

We can boost the circulation with drugs that stimulate
the heart and improve blood flow to the kidneys and
though this may work temporarily, there is little we can do
to make dead muscle work again. As mentioned, prompt
medical attention and the use of clot-busting drugs as early
as possible can prevent too much damage occurring.
Younger patients with cardiogenic shock may end up having a heart transplant.

Heart failure

If patients with extensive damage to the heart muscle survive, the two major complications are heart failure and
rhythm disturbances.

The medical definition of heart failure is difficult to
translate. Imagine you are driving a Rolls-Royce when suddenly its engine is replaced by that of a lawnmower! It just
cannot cope. Heart failure produces breathlessness, ankle
swelling, fatigue, loss of muscle strength and can be totally
disabling. The patient will usually need to take many medications which may have side-effects such as headaches or
sickness. Depression is understandably common in someone who one minute was fit and the next partially or
totally disabled.

When the pumping function of the heart is defective or
if the left inlet valve leaks, a traffic jam of blood forms,
queuing to get back into the heart to be pumped around
the body. The heart has to pump out what it receives, but if
the muscle is damaged the pumping chamber (ventricle)
may not clear efficiently and the pressure in the left filling
chamber (atrium) rises. This pressure rise is transmitted all
the way back into the veins which take blood from the
lungs. When under pressure, the water in blood is forced

out; it flows into the air sacs in our lungs (which are normally quite dry) and congests them, just as water running into a bath will overflow if the bath cannot empty.

If this is only mild the patient may have no symptoms, although congestion of the lungs may be apparent on the chest x-ray. If it is severe, the patient may have to work hard to get the breath in and out of the lungs and will become breathless. At its most severe, the patient may cough up frothy fluid from the air sacs.

To understand what the lungs look like, examine a bath sponge. The holes in the lattice of the sponge can be thought of as the air sacs. When the sponge is dry you can squeeze it without much effort, and it will compress easily. If you now soak the sponge in the bath and make it waterlogged it takes much more effort to compress the sponge; this increased effort is the same for the lungs and is one of the reasons why people feel breathless. The jargon for lungs filling up with water is *pulmonary oedema* (*pulmonary* means 'lung' and *oedema* (pronounced er-deem-er) means 'fluid'). This can be serious, because when the lungs are waterlogged, they cannot transfer oxygen and carbon dioxide as efficiently as they normally do. Sometimes, people who have suffered a heart attack have one bout of pulmonary oedema which, once treated with medication, does not recur.

Rhythm disturbances

A further complication of a damaged heart can be an unstable rhythm. Transient rhythm disturbances are common in the first day or so, even with a mild heart attack, but more serious rhythm disturbances, a sudden awareness of the heart beating, dizziness or fainting, may need treatment with powerful rhythm-controlling drugs. These may have severe side-effects, so careful monitoring is required.

Sometimes, instead of going too fast the heart beats too slowly, because the 'electrical wiring' system may also be damaged during the heart attack. In these circumstances an artificial pacemaker may be needed. Rhythm disturbances and pacemakers are covered in more detail in Chapter 6.

If having read this last section you have become paranoid and depressed, let me reassure you that with proper assessment and treatment, the majority of heart attack victims can get back to normal. Apart from high-technology investigations which are desirable, but not always available, attention to lifestyle and risk factors is vital. Patients need to know how much they can do, such as when they can start driving again, when they can resume normal sexual relations and, in some cases, when they can get back to work. The quality of advice certainly varies and I can recall seeing in one handbook the phrase: 'If you feel sexually aroused, please ring your doctor.' Very few of my patients have followed this advice, and long may that tradition continue! I usually tell patients that they can resume normal sexual relationships, 'home' matches being better than 'away' ones!

Some years ago a few researchers with obviously too little to do studied which position was best for heart attack sufferers to use for sex – street gossip had it that the missionary position was less of a strain for a man with a damaged heart ... I do not suppose there was a shortage of volunteers for this study, although how on earth they were supposed to peform normally while all sorts of measurements were being made at the same time I cannot imagine!

AFTER A HEART ATTACK

So what should happen to a patient after a heart attack,

uncomplicated or complicated? There are two main factors which can decide this: the attitude of the physician looking after the patient, and the resources available.

Dealing with attitude first, you will find, at one end of the spectrum, the conservative doctor who will dispense advice regarding smoking and lifestyle and will do very little else. At the other end of the spectrum is the cardiologist who will want to use all the investigations available to try and work out the patient's risk. By risk, I mean the likelihood of some future problem such as another heart attack, severe rhythm disturbance, heart failure or even sudden death. There would clearly be no point in collecting this information if we felt there was nothing we could do about it but, fortunately, in many cases we can identify patients who are at high risk, and either give medical treatment or carry out a surgical procedure to lower the risk. None of our tests is perfect, and the heart in particular can be unpredictable. The one piece of equipment that you cannot buy at a medical suppliers is a crystal ball!

In the uncomplicated heart attack patient, the questions we need to answer are:

1 Is there a risk of another clot forming in the same artery?
2 How much damage has been done to the muscle?
3 Are the other coronary arteries all right or are they significantly narrowed as well?

To deal with the questions in order:

There is no perfect test to help us decide whether a clot is going to re-form in the same place. Most people do not form a second clot once they have left hospital, but a minority of patients do form a second blood clot, but currently there is little we can do to predict it. So all heart specialists are in the same boat as far as this question is concerned. Where opinons differ is in the attitude to the questions of damage to the heart muscle and to the coronary arteries.

It is usually obvious from a thorough physical examination whether the heart has been severely damaged or not. If the pulse rate is not too fast and the blood pressure is well maintained and if the chest x-ray shows clear lungs, it would seem that the damage is slight, or at least not enough to impair the circulation. The more active cardiologist might organise a scan to look at the heart's function. This can either be done with ultrasound (echo scan) or using a small amount of radioactivity. These tests are described in Chapter 9.

The main question in the case of an uncomplicated heart attack is whether the other coronary arteries are narrowed? Here attitudes will differ from doctor to doctor. Although there are obviously exceptions, the younger generation of specialists often have a more enquiring attitude than older ones. Attitudes may also be linked to the resources available and to specialist workload, as well as to any individual prejudices. A heart specialist who works in a hospital without easy access to some of the more high-tech investigations may well be forced to adopt a more conservative approach, particularly so if he or she has a large number of heart attack patients. Some will not undertake any *prognostic testing* at all (by prognostic, I mean attempting to predict the future), because they are so inundated with work that they are only able to undertake further investigations in people who have symptoms (such as recurrent angina pain after a heart attack) and not do anything for a patient who, on the surface, appears well.

Others will have an age cut-off at perhaps 65 or 70. For example, someone over the age of 65 who has no symptoms may not have access to prognostic testing, whereas someone under the age of 65 will. It is difficult to defend this 'ageism', as the numbers on a birth certificate may have very little to do with a person's physical and mental condition and quality of life. The principle that prognostic testing and the correction of any serious defects should depend on age alone is, in my view and in the view of many of my colleagues, untenable.

People may deny that rationing of care exists. But it clearly does and is often based on such arbitrary cut-off points. However, doctors who know they must handle hundreds of patients per year have to make some difficult decisions. Additionally, if there are long waiting-lists for the tests wanted, specialists may be deterred from adding to the queue. (This can be especially true if the doctor receives menacing letters from the Trust Hospital Management, saying that unless the 'long-waiters' are dealt with the hospital will incur fines under the Patient's Charter!)

A year ago, a friend of mine received a letter from a manager informing him that he had five patients who had been waiting more than eighteen months for treatment, that this was unacceptable and what did he propose to do about it? He just cancelled five other patients without telling them why and dealt with the long-waiters instead even though they were less urgent. What a way to run a chip shop!

Specialists who have access to high technology will find many fewer obstacles to investigating patients and therefore may be less inclined to set age limits. At the very least, any patient who is considered biologically fit should be asked to undergo a treadmill or walking test after a heart attack. This might be followed up by a special x-ray dye test of the arteries (called an *angiogram* or arteriogram). If heart specialists were put on oath, most of the modern generation would agree that an angiogram should be carried out on otherwise fit people who have had a heart attack. But because angiograms are not universally available, we use the treadmill test to decide who is the most deserving.

The treadmill test is thus the poor man's angiogram. Because treadmill tests are cheaper than angiograms and do not involve the use of hospital beds or expensive technology, more of these can be carried out in the NHS. However, treadmill tests may show abnormalities even if the patient has no symptoms.

In the patient who has had a more complicated heart attack the treatment will be different. If there is a plumbing problem, such as a leaking valve, this may be dealt with surgically. The majority of complicated heart attacks involve those where a large amount of healthy heart muscle has been destroyed, so treadmill tests may not have much relevance in predicting what the future holds. From research carried out in the last twenty years or so, we know that the damage to the heart is the most important predictor of the future. In other words, if the heart is severely damaged the number of narrowed arteries may not be too important.

I do not want to give the impression that such patients are written off by their specialists, because much effort has gone into looking at ways of improving survival in people with damaged hearts. These are covered in Chapter 10.

SECURING THE BEST TREATMENT

I hope that those of you who have had heart attacks will feel slightly more informed than you have previously been, and perhaps those destined to have a heart attack in the future will feel more confident about what questions to ask, so that you will not be fobbed off with inadequate explanations. Perhaps the following sample exchange with a patient six days after a heart attack might be of help.

CONSULTANT: Good morning, Mr Hickson. I am Dr

Barford. How are you feeling?

PATIENT: Very well, doctor, thank you.

CONSULTANT: Well, as you have been told by my registrar, you have had a heart attack involving the back wall of the heart. But everything seems fine now.

PATIENT: Er, thank you, doctor. I know that I was given a clot-buster drug when I came in. But how do you know that it has worked?

CONSULTANT: It's difficult to say. There are some changes on your ECG, but they may be less severe than they would have been if you had not had the clot-buster drug.

PATIENT: But I have read that without doing certain tests, it is not possible to say what the future holds.

CONSULTANT: What, exactly, do you mean?

PATIENT: Well, is there any evidence that my heart has been severely damaged and, if so, how badly? Am I going to be able to lead a normal life?

CONSULTANT: Certainly, we have no reason to believe that your heart has been very badly damaged. Your lungs are not congested. Your blood pressure is good, and you have had no more pain since.

PATIENT: How do I know that I am not going to have another heart attack? I understand that I have to modify my lifestyle, stop smoking, which I have already done, and lose some weight. But, aren't there some tests I should go through?

CONSULTANT: It's quite difficult to predict whether you are going to have another heart attack or not. You are on aspirin, which you will need to take long term, and this helps to stop little blood clots forming. We have also put you on a beta-blocker which protects the heart.

PATIENT: Yes, I read that too. The other doctor mentioned something about a treadmill test at some stage in the future.

CONSULTANT: That's right, we like patients under a certain age to have treadmill testing. But it is not our policy to do this with patients over 65. And you are, let's see, 67.

PATIENT: So what! I am still working, I've never been ill before this and I have two small grandchildren. I want to know, as accurately as possible, what my future holds. Are you telling me that I cannot have a treadmill test, at the very least?

CONSULTANT: We only have limited resources available, Mr Hickson. And if we did these tests on everyone, we would be completely snowed under with work. We have to set priorities.

PATIENT: Yes, doctor, I understand your problems. And I have seen how difficult it is for you to cope in this hospital. After all, I did spend several hours on a trolley in casualty. You are talking about my life, however, and I am entitled to have the same tests as anybody else, aren't I?

CONSULTANT: Well, I suppose you are very fit. It would be reasonable to carry out a treadmill test, in a month or two, and we will see what it shows.

PATIENT: And then, if the treadmill test is abnormal, will I get the x-ray dye test of my arteries?

CONSULTANT: Well, probably if you only get symptoms on the treadmill, such as more chest pain.

PATIENT: I am sorry to keep going on, doctor, but I read in a book on heart attacks that it is possible for the treadmill test to show changes that might be important, even if I don't get any pain. Is that right?

CONSULTANT: Well ... er ... that's right.

PATIENT: So, in other words, you are saying that I could have an abnormal treadmill test, but you aren't going to do anything about it. That does not make sense.

CONSULTANT: Look, Mr Hickson, it really is no fun for us having to practise medicine in a situation where you have to constantly think about resources. In an ideal world, you would obviously have all the tests available. Unfortunately, this is not an ideal world.

PATIENT: I appreciate that, doctor. But I have only got one life and I want to hang on to it. So, would you please organise the x-ray dye test of my arteries for me? I don't care if I have to wait a few months, but I read in this book that if I only have one artery blocked my future is very good, but if all the other arteries are furred up I might need an operation. Isn't that true?

CONSULTANT: Well, yes it is. Thank goodness all my patients aren't as well-informed as you, otherwise my life would be impossible! (Turns to his registrar) Let's organise an angiogram for Mr Hickson.

PATIENT: Thank you, doctor.

The purpose of this interview is not to show anybody in a bad light, but merely to make the point that if you are informed about what sort of treatments are available, you are more likely to get them than if you remain ignorant and allow the system to do you down.

4

DOORS THAT JAM ...
VALVE DISEASE

In Chapter 1 I described the heart valves as being like doors which let blood in and out of chambers of the heart. When they are healthy, they only permit blood to go in one direction. There are four valves – an inlet and outlet valve on the right side of the heart and an inlet and outlet valve on the left side.

The valves consist of tissue called *cusps* or *leaflets* which are normally thin, like leaves of a tree. Three of the valves have three cusps, while the inlet valve on the left side only has two. This valve is called the *mitral valve* because when the two cusps are together they resemble an archbishop's mitre. To get some idea of how it works, put your hands together, as if in prayer, but do not interlock your fingers. Keeping your thumbs together, do a clapping motion with your hands. When your palms are separated, this is how the valve looks when it is open, and when they are together this is how it looks when it is closed.

The valves with three cusps or leaves, when looked at from above, resemble a Mercedes-Benz emblem. The left outlet valve is called the *aortic valve* because it lets blood out of the heart into the main artery or aorta. The right inlet valve is called the *tricuspid valve* (meaning three-leaved) and the right outlet valve, which conducts blood to the lungs, is called the *pulmonary valve* (*pulmonary* meaning 'lung').

People often confuse the coronary arteries with the heart valves; many think that a by-pass operation involves 'changing their valves'. However, the valves are separate from the arteries, which supply blood to the heart muscle. The diagram of blood flow through the heart on page 16 shows the position of each of the valves and their names.

Most of the common diseases affect the left-side valves. Diseases of these valves can either be congenital (meaning present at birth) or, more commonly, can be acquired from diseases contracted during a person's life. Sometimes congenital valve disease is part of a more complex disease process, involving the whole heart. As congenital heart disease is a complex subject, beyond the scope of this book, I will concentrate mainly upon acquired disease.

There are only two things that can go wrong with a valve. It can either become blocked, thereby obstructing the flow of blood going through it, or it can leak and let blood flow backwards as well as forwards. Valves become blocked or leak in the same way as valves in an engine or a central heating system. The jargon for an obstructed valve is *stenosis* and for a leaking valve is *regurgitation* or *incompetence*.

OBSTRUCTED VALVES (STENOSIS)

What makes a valve become obstructed? There are many causes, and some valves are more commonly affected than others.

Right outlet (pulmonary) valve

The pulmonary valve is most commonly narrowed at birth. This is called *pulmonary stenosis* and may be an isolated defect, or associated with other abnormalities. There is a congenital defect with the wonderful name of *Tetralogy of*

Fallot. (It sounds like something you see through a telescope in the night sky, but in fact, *tetralogy* just means 'foursome' and Fallot is the person who described it.) A narrowed pulmonary valve is one of the four defects.

Left inlet (mitral) valve

The mitral valve may become narrowed as a consequence of rheumatic fever. This usually occurs in childhood or adolescence so people may not remember having it. It is caused by a common germ called a streptococcus and the first sign of it may be a sore throat, often accompanied by swollen glands in the neck, though not everybody with a streptococcal throat develops rheumatic fever. Rheumatic fever is characterised by joint pains, a skin rash and inflammation of the heart. Sometimes it affects the nervous system and causes involuntary movements called St Vitus' Dance.

The body produces a kind of allergic reaction to the streptococcus, leading to inflammation of the heart and eventually to narrowing of the mitral or other valves (though this may not become apparent until many years after the attack of rheumatic fever). In the era of antibiotics, the disease responds promptly to drugs like penicillin and in any case we see less rheumatic fever now in Europe, since social conditions and hygiene have improved, although it remains common in the Third World. Only about half the patients whose valves show signs of previous rheumatic fever will have had the full-blown disease as a child. Some patients turn up with damaged valves but without knowingly having had rheumatic fever in childhood.

In the case of an obstructed left inlet valve (*mitral stenosis*), the valve will not open properly and the blood finds it difficult to flow from the filling chamber (atrium) into the pumping chamber (ventricle). The pressure in the left atrium therefore rises. This pressure is transmitted back to the lungs, which become congested in a similar way to that described on page 66. However, in this case congestion is not caused through the pump being damaged, but because of a mechanical obstruction (stenosis) to the valve. Stenosis in the valve can be mild, moderate or severe and may progress through these stages as the patient ages. It is not unusual to see a patient who has been well until the age of 50 or 60, and who then develops symptoms. The textbook symptom is breathlessness, occurring at first during vigorous exertion but later on moderate exercise (such as climbing stairs or carrying shopping). In younger women, particularly from Asia or Africa, who are more disposed to mitral stenosis, symptoms might appear for the first time in pregnancy, as the heart has to cope with both the extra weight of a developing baby, and an increased volume of blood because there are now two circulations to deal with.

Because breathlessness may occur during middle age or even later, patients often put their symptoms down to ageing, and fail to seek medical advice. Then, as the obstruction in the valve becomes worse, breathlessness may occur on minimal exertion, such as speaking on the telephone and, typically, when lying flat in bed. This inability to lie flat occurs because the lungs become congested, and people may find that they have to sleep with three or more pillows. If, during sleep, the patient slips down the bed, the lungs become congested and the patient wakes up feeling breathless and wants to fling open the window. Such a dramatic symptom is known as *paroxysmal nocturnal dyspnoea* (pronounced dis-pnee-a), which means 'intermittent night-time breathlessness'. This is a fairly late symptom and at this stage people may visit their doctor. I hope that anyone experiencing any breathlessness which seems unusual will go and consult their doctor.

79

One of the consequences of the pressure rising in the left filling chamber (atrium) because of the valve being obstructed is that the atrium becomes swollen. A change in the heart's rhythm may then occur, and this may cause symptoms to develop for the first time. The upper chambers (atria) stop beating in a coordinated fashion, and start to tremble chaotically at a very fast rate, so that they do not pump blood at all. The textbook description of this, looking at the chambers from the outside, is that they appear to wriggle like a bag of worms! This rhythm disturbance is called *atrial fibrillation* (often shortened to *AF*) and is one of the most common rhythm disorders doctors have to deal with (see Chapter 6 for a more detailed description of fibrillation).

Left outlet (aortic) valve

The aortic valve can also be damaged by rheumatic fever although it would be more likely to leak than narrow. Such damage often accompanies damage to the left inlet (mitral) valve. Certain conditions do cause the aortic valve to narrow, the commonest one being old age. People in their 70s or 80s or sometimes even earlier may form a layer of chalk over the delicate cusps of the valve. This results in the valve becoming rigid until eventually it may not open properly.

Unlike damage to the mitral valve, it is possible to have severe narrowing of the aortic valve with no symptoms at all. This does not mean that it should be ignored, because aortic valve narrowing (stenosis) is potentially lethal. Symptoms only develop at a late stage, the three most typical being heart pain (angina), shortness of breath and sudden blackouts. Again, because these are often put down to old age, they may be overlooked and it is important that any patients displaying such symptoms should have their hearts listened to for a narrowed aortic valve.

The language barrier can often throw up some amusing incidents. I say this with the greatest respect and affection for all the numerous foreign doctors I have worked with in hospitals throughout my career. We had one doctor from China who, although extremely bright, simply could not pronounce the word 'valve'. He had seen some of our patients a few times in the outpatient clinic and after he had returned home, I saw one of these patients for a six-monthly check-up. The conversation went like this:

ME: Good afternoon, Mr Smythe. How have you been? I see you have come for a check-up on your narrowed aortic valve.

MR SMYTHE: No, doctor, there is nothing wrong with my valves. I've got a narrowed wow.

ME: I beg your pardon?

MR SMYTHE: Like I said, I have a narrowed wow!

ME: There is no such thing as a narrowed wow.

MR SMYTHE: Well, I have been told on my last three visits here that I have a narrowed aortic wow, and it hasn't changed!

A quick skim through the notes revealed that Mr Smythe had been seen by the doctor from China on the last three visits and had faithfully believed, and no doubt told his family, that he had an 'abnormal aortic wow'!

Sometimes symptoms occur in younger people, often because the valve only develops with two cusps, instead of three. These valves are described as *congenitally bicuspid* and may be found in patients of any age. It is possible for valves to work normally like this for many years, though they may be likely to wear out prematurely.

Whatever the cause, a narrowed aortic valve means that the heart muscle has to pump blood through a smaller opening, and therefore has to work much harder. In the same way that the biceps and chest muscles will get larger if you lift weights on a regular basis, so the heart muscle will become thicker if it has to work harder. A thickened heart muscle may function normally, but eventually the muscle has to work so hard that it may become fatigued and damaged, and may stretch or dilate. If this happens, even changing the valve surgically may not necessarily cause the heart to shrink to its normal size. However, even if someone with severe aortic narrowing has no symptoms, doctors advise that the valve should be surgically changed. I will discuss how we assess the severity of a narrowed valve later.

LEAKING VALVES

When heart valves are not narrowed, but leak instead, blood goes backwards and the one-way street rule is broken. Leaks in the right outlet (pulmonary) valve are usually not very important, but leaks in the left-side valves are.

Rheumatic fever can cause the valve cusps to become thickened and distorted, so that not only do the doors fail to open, but they do not shut properly either. It is possible to have a valve which is not only obstructing, but also leaking at the same time.

Left inlet (mitral) valve

A leaking mitral valve may also be caused by a heart attack when the valve or its attachments are damaged. It might also occur, out of the blue, when part of the attachment of the valve breaks or ruptures, but this is rare. The valve is attached to the wall of the heart's pump by a series of complicated muscles called *papillary muscles* and related rope-like structures called *chordae* (pronounced kor-dee). Imagine such a muscle as the body of a squid, with the chordae as its tentacles. When these tentacles rupture, the valve starts to leak.

How ill a patient becomes when the valve leaks depends both on its cause and on how quickly the leak develops. If the leak accompanies a major heart attack, the patient may be desperately ill, but if the leak is caused by rheumatic fever, it may take several years before it produces symptoms. The heart uses several mechanisms to compensate for the leak. For example, the left-side filling chamber (atrium) will expand to accommodate the leak, just like a balloon being blown up slowly. The main pumping chamber (left ventricle) may also expand gradually and the muscle may thicken. A person may have a leaking mitral valve for a long time and never feel bad with it. On the other hand, if a leak develops suddenly, and the atrium has no time to expand, the lungs may suddenly fill with water, and the patient may even die. Spontaneous rupture of the squid-like tentacles can also occur, but this is rare.

Finally, I should mention the condition known as the *floppy mitral valve syndrome*. This has several other names, including *mitral valve prolapse* or *Barlow's syndrome*, named after the professor who discovered it. Although extremely common, this condition is often the cause of much needless anxiety to patients. It is often picked up on routine examination, and experienced stethoscope users will hear the tell-tale signs of a clicking noise or peculiar murmur. These may come and go, so that they are audible one day but not the next.

In this condition the valve is floppy and the squid-like tentacles which attach it to the heart muscle may be slack, like loose guitar strings. Although the condition usually produces no symptoms, people can be alarmed when a doctor, listening to their heart, starts to frown and make umming and ahhing noises. Rest assured that in the vast majority of cases the condition is compatible with a totally normal life. There are some associated symptoms, such as odd chest pains or cardiac rhythm disturbances (described in Chapter 6). These symptoms such as a thumping heart or the sensation of missed beats are generally not serious, but occasionally they may need treatment because they cause unpleasant symptoms. Very rarely, floppy mitral valves may leak and become progressively worse with time, but this is not the rule.

Patients with a suspected floppy valve will usually be studied by the echo scan technique. If the diagnosis is proven, patients should always be advised to tell their dentist, obstetrician, etc that they have a floppy heart valve, because even a mild abormality like this can put the patient at risk from the valve becoming infected (see below). However, one should not be disabled because a heart valve is floppy.

Left outlet (aortic) valve

The aortic valve may leak for reasons other than rheumatic fever. Such reasons include diseases of the joints and even inflammation of the bowel. Sometimes, usually in people with high blood pressure or with abnormality of the body's tissues, the aorta may tear spontaneously, making the valve leak. This is a rare but serious illness known in jargon as a *dissection* or *dissecting aneurysm*. When the aortic valve leaks, it increases the volume of the heart's main pumping chamber (ventricle). The consequence depends on how quickly this takes place. With a gradually worsening leak (like that found in rheumatic fever), the ventricle may expand to accommodate the extra volume and no symptoms will develop for many years. Only when the ventricle cannot accommodate the extra blood any longer does it fail to pump properly and symptoms of shortness of breath develop.

When the aortic valve leaks suddenly, the left ventricle finds itself overwhelmed with the extra volume of blood and cannot cope. This leads to the lungs becoming congested and to a seriously ill patient.

Right inlet (tricuspid) valve

I have not yet said much about this valve. It can also be damaged in the same way as the others, by rheumatic fever, but much less dramatically. The main problem with this is that it can leak. Most usually this happens when the right pumping chamber (ventricle) becomes stretched or enlarged, causing the tricuspid valve to stretch too. The right ventricle becomes enlarged when the pressures in the lungs go up and the commonest cause of this is when the left ventricle is severely damaged. However, the pressure in the lungs can also go up when the left inlet (mitral) valve is diseased and a leaking tricuspid valve often accompanies mitral valve disease. When the tricuspid valve leaks, the right-side filling chamber (atrium) stretches and distends even more, so that the pressure in all the veins around the body (but not the veins in the lungs) goes up.

Just as the lungs fill up with water when the mitral valve leaks, when the tricuspid valve leaks, water is forced out into the lining of the abdominal organs or intestines. This accumulation of water can cause the abdomen to distend, making it look as if the patient has suddenly become fat or pregnant. This condition of water in the lining of the intestinal organs is called *ascites* (pronounced ass-eye-tees).The other typical place where water accumulates is around the ankles and legs. People may notice that their ankles become so swollen they cannot get their shoes on, and that if they press the skin of their legs it leaves a pit where the water has been squeezed. Water in the tissues due to a leaking tricuspid valve can be regarded as veins overflowing and flooding the surrounding tissues. Severe fluid retention is a consequence and people may accumulate several litres of fluid in their tissues and gain weight accordingly.

INFECTED VALVES (ENDOCARDITIS)

One other condition which can cause a sudden catastrophic leak in a valve is when the valve becomes infected. Infection of a heart valve is called *endocarditis* (jargon for 'infection inside the heart'). This is not the same as rheumatic fever, where damage to the valve occurs a long time after the bacterial infection. In endocarditis, bacteria find their way into the bloodstream, settle on a valve and start to destroy it.

This condition usually occurs in a valve which is already in some way abnormal, for example, in an aortic valve which has two cusps instead of three, in a valve previously damaged by rheumatic fever or in a floppy valve. Normally the body's defences kill the bacteria before they can do any harm, but in certain people with damaged valves endocarditis can occur. The usual source of these bacteria is from the teeth and it is not uncommon for patients with endocarditis to have been to the dentist some four to six weeks previously. We all have bacteria in our mouths which enter our bloodstream even when we brush our teeth. However, as we are not all dropping like flies from endocarditis, maybe the development of the illness has something to do with our resistance to infection.

Endocarditis normally affects the left-side valves, but in certain people, particularly intravenous drug abusers, infection can be introduced into the veins by dirty needles and settle on the right-side valves – it does not matter which vein such drug abusers use as all these veins drain into the right side of the heart. You can imagine how easy it is for germs to get into the bloodstream when dirty water or dirty needles are used.

Endocarditis usually develops slowly and is characterised by loss of appetite, a general feeling of being unwell, intermittent or continuous temperature and weight loss. These symptoms can, of course, occur in many other conditions but endocarditis should be at the front of a doctor's mind in somebody with signs of an abnormal heart valve. Patients who know they have an abnormal valve should certainly seek medical advice if an illness like this develops.

Even in this age of antibiotics endocarditis is still a grave illness requiring prompt treatment. Although endocarditis usually develops slowly, it can sometimes be a more dramatic illness, where the bacteria destroy the valve very quickly. It is crucial for doctors to diagnose endocarditis quickly and start treatment with the right antibiotics to kill the infection. This can mean a stay in hospital of up to six weeks or longer, and treatment will often require replacement of the valve with an artificial one.

DIAGNOSING VALVE DISEASE

How do doctors diagnose heart valve disease? The patient's symptoms may offer a clue, but the physical examination is also vital. Often, the doctor will inspect the veins in the neck (called the *jugular veins*) and look for the typical rise and fall of blood in these veins. The liver may also become distended in certain circumstances and cause pain in the right side of the abdomen, and indeed this condition can be mistaken for gallstones.

The pulse felt in the wrist or the neck may be abnormal, and leaking or obstructed valves produce funny noises in the heart called *heart murmurs* which have baffled generations of medical students. A murmur is basically a musical noise coming from the heart. It is not a symptom or a diagnosis. No one ever dies of a heart murmur, just as they never die of a floppy valve!

Despite this, some people believe that once having been diagnosed as having a heart murmur, they are seriously ill and try to use it to their benefit. A friend and I overheard a conversation in a restaurant in California, where a middle-aged man proudly announced: 'Since I have been diagnosed as having a systolic heart murmur, which has been proven on echo scanning, I have to take life much easier. I don't have to do any household chores any more!'

The noise is caused by blood flowing through a chamber in a slightly turbulent manner; it is rather like the noise from a choppy sea, while a calm sea is silent. If you put your ear next to a radiator when the heating is on, you will hear a soft whooshing noise as water flows through it. This is similar to a murmur. Many people have heart murmurs who have nothing wrong with their hearts, and these are called innocent murmurs. Approximately 90 per cent of patients referred to hospital with a murmur will have innocent ones. Murmurs can be present in perfectly healthy people, and be compatible with a long and healthy life.

There are two types of heart murmur: those that occur during the contraction phase of the heartbeat (*systolic murmurs*) and those that occur during the relaxation of the heart, while it is filling (*diastolic murmurs*). Systolic murmurs are more common, and the vast majority of them are innocent. Diastolic murmurs are generally more difficult to hear and are always abnormal. Obstructions to flow often produce loud murmurs, like the hissing noise from a kink in a garden hose.

There is a story of an elderly specialist who was trying to teach a group of medical students about a heart murmur. When none of the students could hear it, despite repeated attempts, the consultant announced: 'This murmur is so obvious, I could hear it through nineteen blankets! Sister – please bring nineteen blankets.' Sister duly fetched nineteen blankets (in those days, they tended to obey the doctors to the point of being servile!). At the consultant's behest, she piled the nineteen blankets on top of the terrified patient. The consultant then climbed up onto a stool, dropped the bell of his stethoscope on top of the nineteenth blanket, and pronounced in Gielgudian tones: 'There you are – clear as a bell!'

Attitudes have changed since then and I can just imagine what would happen if I tried to pull such a stunt! It is likely that I would be gently, but firmly, escorted off the ward by men in white coats!

The black magic of heart murmurs could also be used to score points off colleagues. There was once a professor who liked to turn up on his colleagues' ward rounds and impress them with his knowledge of basic science. He would always know the latest publications, and express surprise when his colleagues did not know as much as he did. One eminent heart specialist decided to get his own back. When the know-it-all professor turned up on his ward round, the heart specialist invited him to listen to a patient's heart murmur in order to compare findings. The conversation went something like this:

HEART SPECIALIST: You will, no doubt, hear the rumbling murmur of a stenosed mitral valve.

PROFESSOR:	(listening intently with his stethoscope) Yes, yes! I do believe I can hear that.
HEART SPECIALIST:	Do you also agree that the first heart sound is louder than normal?
PROFESSOR:	Yes, I would agree that the first heart sound is definitely loud.
HEART SPECIALIST:	And, no doubt, you can hear the opening snap that precedes the rumbling murmur.
PROFESSOR:	Yes, there is a typical opening snap!
HEART SPECIALIST:	So you agree, then, that this lady shows the typical signs of mitral stenosis.
PROFESSOR:	Yes, absolutely!
HEART SPECIALIST:	Oh, wait a minute. This is not Mrs Jones! My mistake. This lady does not, of course, have mitral stenosis, but has a totally normal heart. Next patient, sister.

The red-faced professor was not so keen to show off in future!

Previous generations of heart specialists had very little to do apart from listen to whizzes and squeaks inside the heart and pontificate about them. Nowadays if a doctor is not sure about a murmur it does not really matter because the heart can be examined in the same way as the baby developing in the mother's womb, using ultrasound scanning. Suspected valve narrowings or leakages can be examined in this way and the scans will show whether or not the valve is thickened, covered in a chalky deposit, or distorted in any way.

It is also possible to look at the speed at which blood flows through a valve and in which direction it travels. The combined visualisation of a valve and the measurement of the speed and direction of the blood is known as an echo-Doppler scan. The Doppler effect is the phenomenon when a police car, ambulance or fire engine screams past you and the tone of the siren changes as the vehicle speeds away. The same principle can be harnessed to look at damaged heart valves and helps assess the severity of a valve narrowing or leak.

Innocent heart murmurs are usually fairly obvious by the way they change when the patient breathes in, sits up or lies down. The ECGs will usually be normal, and if there is any doubt an echo scan can be carried out. It is advisable to do an echo scan in anybody with a heart murmur because this will show whether there is any structural abnormality. If there is not there is no need to take precautions against infection of the valve (endocarditis). It also provides confirmation, should it be required, that the patient is normal from the point of view of life assurance. If the murmur is not innocent, the doctor may see certain changes on the ECG or the chest x-ray. The echo-Doppler scan, though, is still the most effective technique for assessing abnormal heart valves.

Once the clinical examination and initial tests such as the echo scan have been completed, a heart specialist should have some idea of what is wrong, if anything. The specialist has to decide whether to do something about the valve or just observe it. The action will depend on not only how severe the problem is but also on which valve is involved, as explained earlier.

With a leaking left inlet (mitral) valve, a cardiologist would certainly consider replacing the valve if the patient is severely breathless, or if the main pumping chamber (left ventricle) shows signs of being under excessive strain. If the leak is not that severe, or is well tolerated, surgery may not be required. Obviously, when a leaking mitral valve occurs suddenly, such as after a heart attack, or when one of the squid-like tentacles break, surgery is virtually inevitable.

A left outlet (aortic) valve can also have a severe leak with no symptoms. If the pump function of the heart remains normal, and the heart shows no sign of swelling, we may leave well alone, and follow the patient up at six-monthly or annual intervals.

Patients being considered for surgery will usually need to undergo the x-ray dye test described in Chapter 9, although this test will be assessed in a different way, to measure the pressures in the chambers around the valve to get an idea of the obstruction, or to look at the flow of dye backwards through a leaking valve.

Patients who are advised to continue without surgery will still need their valves listened to and perhaps scanned by echo once or twice a year to monitor any progression. They will also need to report to their doctor any change in symptoms that occur in the intervening period. This is in order to monitor conditions that may be slowly progressive.

A *pressure gradient* is used to assess narrowed valves. This gradient can be measured either by the echo scan or by measuring pressures either side of the valve directly. When a valve is working normally, the pressure on either side will be the same when it is open. If a valve becomes obstructed, the pressure in front of it goes up in relation to the pressure behind the valve, and this difference is called a gradient. The worse the obstruction, the higher the gradient. Thanks to the echo-Doppler scan, we can monitor these gradients quite easily.

TREATMENTS FOR VALVE DISEASE

What treatments can we offer patients with narrowed or leaking heart valves? If surgery is not required, tablets will be given to try and reduce congestion of the lungs, or if the valve is leaky, to open up the arteries in the body to encourage less blood to leak backwards and more blood to go forwards.

There are several medicines available to doctors to achieve these goals. Nowadays, many doctors would use the ACE inhibitors, described in Chapter 10, combined with diuretics (or water pills). In some cases, where the upper chambers have gone out of rhythm (fibrillation), drugs may be given to slow the heartbeat. The most common one is called digoxin. However, everyone is different, so if you have a valve problem and you are not on one of these medications, please do not go waving a copy of this book at your doctor and insist that he change your treatment! Sometimes the problem is so mild that no tablets are needed.

If surgery is required, a narrowed or blocked valve can be split open. If this cannot be achieved, the valve can be replaced. Similarly, it may be possible to repair a leaking valve, although in most cases it will need to be replaced.

Recently, a new technique has been developed which allows heart specialists to split mitral valves open from the outside, with the patient awake. This is particularly useful in young patients, where the valve has not become covered with a layer of chalk, and where the attachments of the valve (i.e. the tentacles of the squid-like structure) are in good condition. Results in these patients can be spectacular.

Much work goes into deciding which patients are suitable for this technique, which nowadays means having a different type of echo scan. Instead of being carried out from the front of the chest the heart is scanned from behind, in the oesophagus (the gullet or eating tube which connects your mouth to your stomach). To do this, the patient swallows the small echo probe and the pictures of the mitral valve and its attachments are clearer this way. The jargon for this technique is a *trans-oesophageal echo* or *TOE* (which means 'echoing the heart through the gullet').

If everything looks suitable, the procedure is carried out in the same way as most x-ray dye tests are, by accessing the heart and the blood vessels in the right groin. I will not go into the technical details of how one gets a tube from a vein in the leg to the mitral valve, but the procedure is called a *percutaneous mitral valvuloplasty* (a tortuous mouthful which translates as 'altering the shape of the left inlet valve via the skin'). If someone is turned down for this technique, because the valve has been too badly damaged, they will need to have a new valve put in by a heart surgeon.

In the case of a leaking mitral valve, some surgeons do try to repair it if possible, but if it is the aortic valve which is narrowed or leaking, a new valve is necessary. What these operations involve, what their risks are, and what sorts of valve are available will be discussed in Chapter 10.

DIAGNOSING INFECTED VALVES

How do we diagnose endocarditis, or infected heart valves? Apart from the symptoms of general ill health (sweating, loss of appetite, etc), a doctor should be alerted to the possibility of endocarditis by the presence of a heart murmur. There are certain other signs that doctors look for; for example, little lines of bleeding in the nail bed called *splinter haemorrhages*. They look like wood splinters but are small areas of inflammation in the tiny blood vessels or capillaries. The doctor may look for similar signs in the finger pulps or the toes.

The diagnosis is made in two ways. First, samples of blood are taken to see if germs will grow from them (called blood cultures). Several sets of blood culture are taken and microbiologists or bacteriologists will identify the germ and tell the heart specialist which antibiotics to use to kill it.

The second way to reach a diagnosis is to look for infection on the valves. We come back to the trusty old echo scan. Areas of infection often show up as bright spots attached to the valve. These spots are made up of infected material produced by the bacteria attacking the valve, and are called *vegetations* (a jargon word for a growth). Sometimes these vegetations are large, sometimes small. Their progress can be monitored through serial echo scans. They may be well seen on the TOE test, and nowadays we tend to use this sort of echo scan more commonly.

The echo test can also tell us whether the valve is becoming progressively leaky. Remember that endocarditis is one of the causes of a sudden leak in a valve, if the bacteria chew their way through it and cause a hole. If the infection cannot be controlled with antibiotics and particularly if the valve starts to leak dangerously, surgeons must be ready to dive in at any moment and replace it.

Doctors must advise patients with abnormal heart valves to have antibiotic cover before any procedure that might put them at risk from endocarditis (such as dental work, delivery during pregnancy and any operation involving orifices of the body, where bacteria normally lurk!). This is called *antibiotic prophylaxis*. Of course, many people with heart valve abnormalities do have dental treatment and pregnancies without any complications, but if we know that a potential problem exists it is sensible to try and prevent any complications.

Infection in the right inlet (tricuspid) valve is much rarer than infection on the left-side valves, and unlike the left-side heart valves, tricuspid valve endocarditis can be well tolerated. Because of this, although the valve may leak, it is much less common to carry out emergency surgery. The treatment of several weeks of antibiotics is just the same, however.

Now we've seen how to oil the hinges so the doors open and close properly, let's look at the engine!

5

... AND PUMPS THAT PLAY UP
MUSCLE DISEASE

I have described how the heart muscle can be damaged by the loss of its blood supply through coronary artery disease and through becoming stretched and strained by narrowing or leaking valves. Sometimes, however, the heart muscle may be attacked by diseases, even when the arteries and the valves are normal. These diseases are known as disorders of the heart muscle and are called *cardiomyopathies* (*cardio* means heart, *myo* means muscle and *pathies* means disease). This term should only be applied to diseases where no obvious secondary causes (such as impaired blood flow or valve disease) exist.

There are three different kinds of muscle disorder, two of which are relatively common, and the third of which is rare and I will therefore only mention in passing.

WEAK PUMPS

The most common muscle disorder occurs when the heart muscle is weakened and fails to contract properly. The effects of this are the same as if the heart muscle had been damaged by a heart attack. This used to be called *congestive myopathy*, because the symptoms were those of congestion. If the left side of the heart is involved the lungs are congested; if the right side is involved the tissues are congested. Where both sides of the heart are damaged, the patient would be both breathless and have swollen ankles.

Nowadays we use the term *dilated myopathy*, where the heart becomes dilated or enlarged. There are various degrees of this condition, ranging from mild impairment with few symptoms to severe impairment where the patient may become very short of breath and cough up frothy liquid from the lungs. The condition may worsen with time.

Sometimes, we can identify certain poisons which can destroy the heart muscle. The commonest identifiable poison is alcohol. Although in small or moderate amounts alcohol makes people feel relaxed and at ease, in large amounts it acts as a poison. The definition of a heavy drinker is difficult, because guidelines vary according to a person's sex and weight. Also, in the medical profession a heavy drinker is usually someone who drinks more than their doctor!

Joking aside, there is no doubt that people who are heavy drinkers or alcoholics run the risk of damaging their heart muscle and ending up with what we call an *alcoholic cardiomyopathy*. Some patients with an extreme form of the condition may end up needing a heart transplant. It is difficult to know why alcohol should affect the heart in this way in some people and not in others. Some doctors have suggested that alcohol is only indirectly responsible and that any heart damage may be due to malnutrition, the connection being that many alcoholics do not eat enough and become vitamin deficient. It is true that some vitamin deficiencies can lead to weakening of the heart muscle. Beri-beri, for example, a condition caused by deficiency of vitamin B, is characterised by a weakness of the heart muscle and heart failure. However, we do see alcoholics who seem to eat well but who nevertheless end up with damaged hearts. If they stop drinking, we sometimes see an improvement in the heart muscle over time.

Other rarer poisons include some heavy metals. For

example, some patients have a rare condition where their bodies become overloaded with iron, and iron deposits occur in the heart muscle which stop it working properly. Other chemicals are also thought to damage the heart. Some years ago I attended a teenage boy who had been glue sniffing. Shortly after, he became severely ill, with fluid pouring out of his lungs, and was transferred to Bart's as an emergency. This young lad had destroyed his heart muscle, developing a dilated myopathy without any other obvious cause and subsequently had a heart transplant.

Although we could not prove conclusively that the glue sniffing had caused the acute illness, it seems too much of a coincidence to assume otherwise. You may have read in the papers accounts of sudden death after glue sniffing. It may be that in certain individuals chemicals in the glue can either cause fatal rhythm disorders or lead to heart muscle destruction. Either way, solvent abuse is a dreadful practice which should be vigorously discouraged and the dangers pointed out.

Sometimes the heart can be damaged shortly after the patient has had a flu-like illness, and has then developed full-blown symptoms of heart failure. Some years ago there was a vogue for doing a test called a *biopsy* in these patients in order to search for inflammation due to viruses in the heart muscle. This entailed pinching out a piece of tissue for examination under the microscope. A heart biopsy is a straightforward procedure carried out using an implement which looks like the jaws of a shark. Unfortunately, try as hard as we may, and even using very high-powered electron microscopes, we have not been able to demonstrate particles of infecting virus in these biopsy tissues.

Inflammation of the heart muscle (called *myocarditis*) is often difficult to diagnose, especially as some low-grade inflammation of the heart muscle accompanies many common viral illnesses. People suffering from a bad dose of flu may show some subtle changes on the ECG during the illness, but a true myocarditis may produce an excessively fast pulse rate and ECG changes.

During the attack of the viral-type illness we think that the heart muscle occasionally becomes permanently damaged. Doctors therefore used to give drugs to counteract the inflammation of a damaged heart. Cortisone, often in quite high doses, was commonly used. Cortisone is a chemical which the body produces to help fight inflammation. We had hoped that these medications would shorten the period of inflammation of the heart muscle and reverse the damage, but unfortunately, they do not seem to work. Patients whose hearts improved seem to have done so in spite of, rather than because of, this treatment. At present, there is little that your doctor can do to prevent this illness. Again, let me put this in perspective. Not everybody who develops a flu-like illness will end up with an irreversibly damaged heart. This remains a rare condition.

Another form of muscle disorder can occur – rarely, thank goodness – in women in the last three months of their pregnancy, or shortly after delivery of the baby. This is called a *peri-partum*, or a *post-partum cardiomyopathy*. These tongue-twisting jargon terms mean 'around the time of delivery' or 'after delivery'. Before you start reaching for the contraceptives, let me stress that I have seen only about half a dozen cases in twenty years. The condition tends to be confined to women over thirty who are on their third or subsequent pregnancy. This muscle disorder is a horrid condition which strikes people down in the prime of life. The exact cause remains a mystery. Some women's hearts will recover spontaneously in the first six to nine months after being diagnosed, whereas others will have damaged hearts and sometimes will need transplants. Partial recovery, where the heart shows some damage but can still cope is also fairly common. Unfortunately, there appears to be very little we can do to reverse the process at the moment.

I have not covered all the conditions which can lead to the heart dilating, but one condition likely to increase is in patients suffering with AIDS. Doctors are beginning to see patients with AIDS-related illnesses whose heart muscles have failed. Again, the exact cause is unknown and, AIDS being a new illness, we are having to learn on our feet.

Most people who have a dilated (enlarged) heart have no identifiable cause for it. When we cannot find a cause for something, we call it *idiopathic*, which simply means that it occurs for an unknown reason. Another word is *cryptogenic*, which means the cause is hidden, like cryptic clues in a crossword.

The treatment of these enlarged, poorly beating hearts will often involve the use of diuretic medicines, which increase the amount of urine the kidneys make and reduce the amount of blood going around, thereby decongesting the lungs and tissues. Sometimes, if the patient is really ill, with low blood pressure, drugs will be given intravenously to try to make the heart beat more strongly. These are called *inotropic drugs* ('inotropic' relates to the force of contraction of the heart). Unfortunately, these drugs only act intravenously, and although they may provide some temporary support, a patient cannot go home attached to a drip for ever. Medicines like digoxin, referred to earlier, may be given, and the ACE inhibitors (see Chapter 10) are also often used, as they have been shown to prolong life in people with damaged hearts.

Patients with such hearts will commonly develop abnormalities of the heart rhythm, some of which can be dangerous or life threatening. The relationship between damaged hearts and rhythm disturbances is described in Chapter 6.

OVER-ENTHUSIASTIC HEARTS

The second most common form of heart muscle disease is a condition where, instead of the heart failing to contract properly, it may contract too vigorously. This condition is characterised by a marked thickening of only one part of the heart muscle, the wall separating the right from the left side of the heart (the septum). Not only does the muscle become thickened, but its structure becomes disorganised and haphazard. This strange condition is known as *Hypertrophic* (meaning 'thickened') *cardiomyopathy* (often abbreviated to HCM and pronounced hocum).

In this condition, the back wall of the heart may be normal or only minimally thickened, whereas the septum may be severely thickened. This condition sometimes runs in families but more usually occurs sporadically. Sometimes it does not produce any symptoms but nevertheless can lead to sudden death. In general it is more serious when diagnosed in childhood or early adulthood, than when it appears in later life. This may just mean that those cases diagnosed in a 50 or 60-year-old were destined not to produce a problem, whereas a catastrophe in a 20-year-old may represent a more aggressive form of the disease. Sometimes the condition is picked up by symptoms such as chest pain, palpitations, dizzy spells or blackouts. Blackouts must be treated seriously, because in HCM rhythm disturbances are common, some of which can be life threatening. Sudden death in this condition is thought to be due to a rapid, irregular rhythm which cannot support the circulation.

In HCM, these rhythm disturbances may occur on exertion. Anyone who feels faint or giddy, or who has a blackout or palpitations during a sporting activity, must be investigated thoroughly.

Sometimes HCM is picked up because the patient will

have an ECG done for some other reason, such as part of a medical for life assurance. The ECG may show changes suggesting that the heart muscle is thickened, or under strain, or show electrical faults. If such abnormalities are found a cardiac echo scan should be carried out. This will usually establish whether the patient has HCM.

How do we treat HCM? If it is picked up at a routine examination and the patient has never had any symptoms or a family history, doctors will be primarily concerned with the electrical stability of the heart. We therefore carry out treadmill tests to see if the heart rhythm is stable on exercise, as well as prolonged monitoring of the heart rhythm while the patient is walking about leading a normal life. In most cases it does not make sense to monitor patients in hospital as we need to know what the heart is doing during ordinary, everyday activity. This can be achieved by wearing a small tape recorder, attached to the belt, which records an ECG for a 24-hour period. Provided these tests are all normal, a HCM sufferer may not require any treatment other than careful follow-up once or twice a year. I will talk more about monitoring the heart rhythm in Chapter 9.

If rhythm disturbances are found, doctors may be forced to give the patient powerful rhythm-controlling drugs. People experiencing abnormalities of rhythm during sporting activity or during an exercise test should be told not to undertake rigorous sport at all. This may mean giving up jogging, tennis or squash. Patients with symptoms such as chest pain may get some relief from groups of drugs like beta-blockers or calcium channel blockers, and powerful rhythm-controlling drugs may be needed (see page 235).

If someone has HCM, it is advisable to screen other members of the family with a clinical examination, an ECG and an echo scan. Some heart specialists have made HCM their life's work and have studied many patients in great detail. In some cases, particularly where children are involved, or in families with a bad medical history, we might re-refer these patients to our colleagues for further advice.

One final word on HCM. As with a floppy mitral valve, if doctors are going to label a patient with a diagnosis, we must make sure that we do not do so too easily. Some doctors use the term HCM fairly loosely in any patient whose echo scan has confirmed a slightly thickened muscle. There are one or two conditions where the heart muscle does show some slight thickening for no apparent reason but it really is not correct to label these people as having 'some sort of hocum'.

The implications of mislabelling someone as having HCM can be devastating. If a GP is asked by a life assurance company or a prospective employer for some medical details and HCM appears, the life assurance or employment may be turned down. So, if you have been diagnosed as having HCM without an echo scan, do please question your doctor as to the validity of the diagnosis. Similarly, if there are members of your family who have unexplained, sudden death, particularly if there is a post-mortem diagnosis which says the words 'cardiomyopathy', it might be advisable to have other members of the family screened, if only to put everybody's mind at rest.

THE HEART IN A STRAITJACKET

The final type of disorder of the heart muscle is rare. This is not one of the heart's ability to contract but an inability to relax. This means that the pressures inside the heart stay high throughout the relaxation phase of the heartbeat, which produces symptoms of breathlessness. It often affects the right-side pumping chamber, so the patient has symptoms of engorgement of the veins, ankle and leg swelling, maybe a tender liver and a swollen abdomen. These disorders are known as *restrictive myopathies*, because the heart is restricted in its capacity to expand properly after each contraction, almost as if the heart was in a straightjacket.

INFLAMMATION OF THE HEART'S LINING (PERICARDITIS)

The lining of the heart (pericardium) may become inflamed after a heart attack. Spontaneous attacks of inflammation of the lining of the heart, known as *pericarditis*, do occur, often in little epidemics and most commonly in young to middle-aged men. We assume it is caused by a virus. The condition may cause pain and a temperature, perhaps with a sore throat and other feelings of ill health. The pain differs from heart attack pain in that it is often made worse by breathing in. Changes in body position, such as sitting up or lying down, will also influence it, whereas in a heart attack, the pain will remain fairly constant.

As an ECG will often show the typical features of pericarditis, the diagnosis can be straightforward. Sometimes the enzymes in the blood, which are released when there is damage to the heart muscle, may also be elevated, which indicates that not only is the lining of the heart inflamed, but that the muscle underneath the lining may be as well. This condition is called *myo-pericarditis*. This is generally a benign condition and usually responds in a few days to conventional anti-inflammatory drugs. A minority of patients will continue to get attacks of *relapsing pericarditis* at varying intervals. Such patients may need to take small doses of cortisone (an anti-inflammatory drug) at certain intervals to make the inflammation settle down. We do not know why this occurs, but it can be disabling and distressing.

Inflammation of the pericardium can occur as part of other rare diseases, particularly conditions where the body's immune system attacks its own organs. It can also occur after a heart operation, because of bruising around the heart which usually lasts a day or so. In some cases, where inflammation of the heart occurs, a layer of fluid collects around the heart. This is called a *pericardial effusion* (*effusion* meaning 'collection of fluid'). Echo scanning will usually show the amount of fluid quite clearly.

Sometimes it is necessary to drain some of the fluid, in the same way that one would drain an inflamed knee. The process, known as a *pericardial tap*, is not usually that difficult and is done under local anaesthetic. Sometimes this tap is done as an emergency because so much fluid has accumulated around the heart that it cannot pump properly.

In the past, one relatively common cause of fluid around the heart was tuberculosis or TB. Infected material would collect around the heart and if not treated properly could make the lining of the heart very thick and full of scar tissue which prevented it from beating properly. This condition, which we see only rarely, is called *constrictive pericarditis*. It is as if the heart is held by a large boa constrictor and struggles to contract and relax properly. In these cases, the treatment is to remove the pericardium surgically, by stripping it away from the heart muscle. Although this type of disease is now rare, we come across the occasional case following major heart surgery, where prolonged inflammation of the lining of the heart have led to the same effects as produced by TB.

CARDIAC TUMOURS

Finally, a word about tumours of the heart muscle.

Tumours can be divided up into those which are *benign* – i.e. do not spread to other parts of the body – and those which are *malignant*, which means they are cancerous and can spread. Tumours are also described as being *primary* or *secondary*. A primary tumour means that is where the tumour has started, and a secondary one is where little seeds of the tumour have spread, either via the bloodstream or through the lymph glands. For example, a heavy smoker may have a primary tumour of the lung but have secondary deposits in the bones and in the liver, or in the brain.

All heart tumours are rare. Secondary tumours, such as from the breast or lung, might infiltrate through the lining of the heart and produce fluid around the heart. Primary heart tumours are even rarer and can be incredibly difficult to diagnose. They might be accompanied by unexplained rhythm disturbances, signs of heart failure, blackouts, unexplained temperatures or even sudden death. Because the tumours often arise from the heart muscle, they may grow and spread, and gradually replace normal heart muscle with cancerous tissue. Such conditions are not necessarily obvious through echo scanning, because they do not stand out, unlike an abnormal shadow on a chest x-ray. Sometimes the diagnosis is therefore made by a heart surgeon from a biopsy (see page 99), or it may not be apparent until after death.

If a tumour is diagnosed, the only real treatment is a heart transplant. This can be successful, because the cancerous growth invading the heart muscle rarely spreads beyond the heart to other organs.

There is one strange tumour which can grow inside the cavity of the heart, usually in the left filling chamber (atrium). This tumour, although benign (i.e. not cancerous) can still be dangerous. This is because as the tumour grows it flops around inside the heart and gets stuck across the left inlet (mitral) valve, effectively causing a blockage, so that circulation stops. This tumour is known as a *left atrial myxoma* (pronounced micksomer). It may be accompanied by fevers and strange sounds when listening to the heart. Bits of the tumour can break off and get stuck in the arterial tree around the body, producing an embolism.

Sometimes certain blood tests become abnormal, although in order to make a diagnosis, you have to suspect a myxoma might be there and look for it. Yes, you have guessed it, this is done with an echo scan, which will show a myxoma as a mass of abnormal echoes near the mitral valve.

The treatment is to remove the myxoma as soon as possible, with a heart operation. What the surgeon usually finds is a tumour attached by a stalk, just like an apple, to the wall of the atrium. This can be removed easily and the patient is cured. No one knows why these strange things develop, but busy heart specialists will usually see one case every year or so. Once they are diagnosed they should be removed immediately in case they obstruct the valve. There is an old adage: 'Never let the sun set on a myxoma.' No doubt this is some relic of the British Empire, but the message is true.

So, enough of pumps, linings and lumps – on to electrical faults and short circuits.

6

THE RHYTHM SECTION
PACEMAKERS AND PALPITATIONS

In normal circumstances the heart's 'battery', the *sinus node*, commands the rate at which the heart beats and keeps the rhythm of the heart regular. We have seen, in Chapter 1, how a wave of activation from the sinus node spreads into the upper chambers (the atria) making them beat. Having travelled through the atria the impulses then converge towards the *atrio-ventricular node* (or *AV node* for short) in the same way that railway tracks converge at a junction. The impulses are held up for a short time by the AV node to allow the atria to finish contracting, before the impulses spread through the lower chambers (ventricles) of the heart giving them messages to contract and pump blood. The sophisticated system of electrical pathways which the sinus node controls can be thought of as the heart's wiring system.

The main pathway below the AV node – the junction – is called the *bundle of His* (pronounced hiss). This divides into three main electrical pathways which travel through the ventricles and are known as *bundle branches*. The *right bundle branch* spreads across the floor of the right ventricle and the *left bundle branch* divides into a front division and a back division. Like the arteries, these bundle branches divide into small electrical pathways which infiltrate through the heart muscle and make it contract.

THE HEART AS A TORTOISE

As with any wiring system, this can go wrong anywhere in

the circuit. If the signals which make the heart contract are held up or blocked at any stage, the messages that tell the heart muscle to beat may not get through and the heart may beat too slowly. Sometimes the heart may even stop for a few seconds and if this happens the patient may feel dizzy or black out. The term for when the heart goes too slowly is *bradycardia*.

If the battery generating the impulses fails the next structure along the pathway recognises that it hasn't had a message and takes over, although it may do so at a slightly slower rate. This fail-safe mechanism operates all the way through the electrical conducting system. The pumping chambers of the heart can even beat without any signals from above. However, we can't rely on them to beat regularly under their own steam and they sometimes stop.

Trouble with the heart's battery

Faults in the electrical conducting system have all been given specific names. For instance, diseases of the heart's battery are known collectively as *sinus node disease*. This covers a wide spectrum of conditions, varying from a slightly slow heart beat to an extreme slowing of the heart and even pauses of several seconds. When the sinus node fails to send out a message an ECG will produce a straight line with no wiggles or bumps. Treatment will depend on whether the patient has any symptoms.

Heart specialists are often referred patients who display slow pulses at routine examination. In these cases a careful medical history must be taken to determine, for example, whether the patient is on any drugs which might slow the heart (such as beta-blocking drugs). Sometimes other conditions such as an under-active thyroid can cause a slow pulse rate. This is because the thyroid gland controls our body's metabolism and the rate at which we turn over various chemicals. If the thyroid gland becomes under-active every process in our bodies slows down, including the heart rate. The doctor will look for typical symptoms such as the patient feeling cold and lethargic, having a change of skin condition, loss of hair and sometimes a deepening of the voice.

Other causes of a slow pulse include athletic training. If you run marathons or do endurance training your body adapts and your tissues become more efficient at extracting oxygen. The heart therefore pumps less rapidly. It is common to find marathon runners with pulse rates of around 40–50 beats a minute; when they are asleep the pulse may drop to 30 beats a minute or less.

Sometimes the sinus node may be temporarily damaged by a heart attack, particularly when the right coronary artery blocks off. If the heart rate slows severely after a heart attack the patient may have a pacemaker wire inserted into a vein in their neck or under the collar bone for a few days. This wire will be attached to a box which may sit on the bedside table and which paces the heart until it recovers its normal function.

Most people with this condition, called *sinus bradycardia*, require no treatment unless there is an underlying condition such as those described above. If someone complains of dizzy spells or faints and a slow pulse is found, some sort of monitoring technique will be used to see if we can detect periods when the heart goes extremely slowly.

Although slow pulse rates often alarm doctors, heart specialists are able to distinguish a normal, slow heart rate from an abnormally slow one caused by disease. One extreme of form of slowing of the heart rate occurs when the nerve that slows the heart is stimulated. In Chapter 1 I discussed a gory play with lots of blood and people faint-ing. Similarly, a young man was admitted to Bart's many years ago with repeated faints. He was fine until someone approached him to take blood but at the sight of the needle his heart stopped beating for several seconds, his eyes rolled up and he collapsed. This is a very extreme form of nerve stimulation and we call it needle phobia. Other phobias, such as fear of spiders (arachnophobia), do not have such a dramatic effect on the heart!

The majority of patients who have true sinus node disease, where the heart beats too slowly or stops at times, have it simply as a consequence of wear and tear. Not surprisingly therefore, it is more common among older people. Even severe slowing of the heart may be well tolerated and not produce any symptoms. Heart specialists have argued for some time about whether artificial heart pacemakers should be put into people who have slow heart rates but no symptoms. It can be quite alarming to see a seven- or eight-second gap on an ECG printout when no heart beat occurs and many heart specialists would be more comfortable if a patient with this condition had a pacemaker implanted.

One strange form of disease of the heart's battery causes the heart to slow down intermittently and in between beat quite fast. The fast rhythms arise from the upper chambers and if we monitor patients for a twenty-four hour period we may see periods of fast heart rate (*tachycardia*), interspersed with periods of slow heart rate. This condition is known as the *tachy-brady syndrome* which is jargon for the fast-slow syndrome – a sort of cardiac foxtrot!

Explaining to patients that sometimes their hearts don't beat fast enough and other times they go too fast is often confusing. After all, how can the heart do both? We had a patient with a rhythm disorder like this on the ward at Bart's. She noticed her heart sometimes beating fast and irregularly and at other times too slowly, and it made her dizzy. Her doctor, trying to explain to her, said: 'Well, dear, the problem is you keep getting a rhythm called fibrillation or flutter and at other times your heart beat goes brady-cardic or too slowly. So tell me, which rhythm suits you best?' She replied brightly: 'Whichever one you say, doctor!'

The problem with treatment is that if we give drugs to stop the heart beating too fast we may make the slow bits worse and vica versa.

Trouble at the junction

The next site at which diseases can cause the heart to go too slowly is at the AV node, or railway junction, where signals coming down from the sinus node via the upper chambers of the heart can be delayed, partially blocked or completely blocked. These diseases are known collectively as *atrio-ventricular block* – often shortened to *AV block*.

If the impulses are simply delayed this will produce no symptoms but will show up on the ECG as a time lag between the upper chambers and the lower chambers beating. This is called *first-degree heart block*. On its own it is of no consequence and is often an incidental finding in people who are otherwise quite well. However, if the impulses are intermittently blocked so that, for example, one beat in every five is blocked, this can be more serious and is known as *second-degree heart block*. Complete heart block, or *third-degree heart block*, means that no impulses get through to the pumping chambers which then have to beat under their own steam.

Both second- and third-degree heart block can occur as isolated abnormalities or as a result of heart attacks. Heart attacks involving the right coronary artery may produce one kind of block whereas those involving one of the left-side arteries can produce a different type. Most commonly, these forms of heart block occur in elderly patients as a result of wear and tear on the electrical system. Sometimes this sort of heart block can occur after major heart surgery,

113

in which case it may be temporary. Some forms of second-degree block require a permanent pacemaker to be implanted; others do not. Complete heart block requires a pacemaker to be implanted.

A bundle of trouble

The bundle branches can also be diseased in a variety of ways, but are commonly found in elderly people as a result of wear and tear. A blocked bundle branch, whether it be a right or left bundle, produces striking abnormalities on the ECG which we have been training medical students (not always totally successfully!) to recognise as a matter of routine.

Right bundle branch block (often known as *RBBB*) can be an isolated finding and doesn't always mean there is something wrong with the heart. Many people live long and healthy lives with this ECG abnormality but they can be unnecessarily frightened by the shake of the doctor's head or the tutting from his lips! Sometimes RBBB can accompany certain congenital heart diseases so it is often sensible to carry out a simple ultrasonic scan of the heart. If the scan is normal and the patient has no other symptoms there is nothing to worry about.

Left bundle branch block (or *LBBB*), on the other hand, is always abnormal, although it is not possible in every case to say why it occurs. It can accompany any disease of the heart muscle or the left-side heart valves or it can follow a heart attack. It is not uncommon to find LBBB in people with HCM (see Chapter 4) or with long-standing high blood pressure. In these cases LBBB may reflect an abnormality of the heart muscle which happens to involve part of the wiring system. The difficulty lies with patients who have no symptoms and no sign of anything else wrong with them but where LBBB is picked up on a routine ECG.

114

I once worked for a wonderful physician who told me: 'Now remember, Duncan, if there was never any indication to do a particular test, you don't have to explain it when it's abnormal.' What he meant was that you shouldn't go around doing routine tests on people who are well because you might find something you have to worry about and need to investigate further. In his many years of experience he had become frustrated by trying to find explanations for every single abnormal test he uncovered. Much of what he said was true.

Today, when health screening is such an important part of doctors' work, we are bound to pick up things we would rather not know about, and unexplained bundle branch block is one of them. We can do a battery of tests and still find absolutely nothing. If you are unfortunate enough to have LBBB it will be difficult for you to obtain life insurance at standard rates. However, if the ECG abnormality is an isolated finding and there is no obvious condition accompanying it, the premium should not be too horrific.

Sometimes combinations of bundle branch blocks occur. Where two of the three bundles are blocked it is known as *bi-fascicular block* (meaning 'two-bundle block'). Sometimes the ECG suggests all three bundles are diseased and this condition is known as *tri-fascicular block*. Patients with bundle branch blocks, especially the elderly, may turn up with dizzy spells or blackouts and this almost certainly means that the heart's electrical pathways fail intermittently and a pacemaker will need to be implanted. I am aware that I may have failed to answer the $64,000 question of 'Why do some people have this abnormality?' but the answer is we just don't know.

PACEMAKERS

What exactly is a pacemaker? It is simply a battery in a

small tin which we implant under the skin. It fires off signals that are conducted down a special wire which has been inserted into the heart. One end of the wire is plugged into the battery and the other end is in contact with the wall of the heart muscle. The signals travelling down the wire make the heart contract.

Pacemaker technology has changed dramatically over the last twenty years. The earliest pacemakers were rather unsophisticated. They were about the size of a sardine tin bulging out from under the skin and their batteries were short lived. Over the years they have become smaller and much more sophisticated and are now about the size of a book of matches. Modern pacemakers can be programmed externally, using a remote control unit like a video recorder's. In this way the pacemaker can be told at what rate it should cut in, how fast it should go and how much electricity it should use; the batteries can also be checked externally. (Nowadays a battery may not need changing for ten years – depending on the use it gets – and this entails a very minor operation.)

The ability of modern pacemakers to recognise the heart's own rhythm is called 'sensing'. There are two circuits in this type of pacemaker: one for sensing the heart's own beat and recognising that it shouldn't put in a paced beat and a second circuit for delivering the beat down the wire. In patients where the heart's wiring has packed up completely the pacemaker will be used all the time. In other patients the heart may slow down or stop only intermittently and the pacemaker will recognise this and cut in to prevent a dizzy spell or blackout. These pacemakers are called *demand pacemakers*. Some really clever pacemakers can actually recognise when their owner is doing something physical and will beat faster under these conditions – these are called *rate responsive pacemakers*.

The most sophisticated pacemakers achieve, as nearly as

possible, the normal sequence of activation of the heart. This is done by using one wire inside the right upper chamber (atrium) and another in the right pumping chamber (ventricle). The two wires are plugged into separate sockets in the pacemaker battery and the atria are paced first, followed by the ventricles. These pacemakers are much more expensive than single-chamber pacemakers where the wire is placed only into the right ventricle.

In an ideal world nearly every pacemaker fitted would be a two-wire, or what we call a *dual chamber pacemaker.* Studies have shown that people generally feel better and more able to lead more active lives when we reproduce the heart's normal functions as closely as possible. Unfortunately, NHS finances don't allow this because these pacemakers are more expensive than the single-chamber ones and we often have to compromise in order to conserve budgets. Many people who should have dual chamber pacemakers may not receive them and this is clearly a form of rationing.

A 95-year-old who is confined to a wheelchair and who keeps blacking out might do very well with a single-chamber pacemaker but anyone who is fit and active should really have the best pacemaker available.

Fitting a pacemaker

Many people think that having a pacemaker implant is a big operation. However, it is not the same as major heart surgery – the operation is usually performed under local anaesthetic and most people only stay in hospital for a day or two. In some instances patients arrive in the morning and go home the same evening.

To put in a pacemaker a cardiologist will use a vein which leads to the right side of the heart. The vein is found near the shoulder joint, or alternatively just under the collar bone, and the area is numbed with a local anaesthetic. If the patient is right-handed the pacemaker is usually put on the left side and vice versa.

The doctor will use an x-ray tube to help him guide the pacemaker wire into the heart and position it appropriately. While this is being done the patient may experience some palpitations or feel the heart thumping strangely. Various measurements are made after a suitable position is found to ensure that the current drain on the battery won't be too great and that the signal of the patient's own heart beat is strong enough to be recognised.

The patient might hear some strange words being used as the doctor converses with the technician. This jargon concerns the electrical signals from the pacemaker so don't be alarmed. One patient, a middle-aged Jewish man with that tongue-in-cheek grumpiness so common in people of his age, had lain still on the operating table during his pacemaker implantation without saying a word. The doctor was just about to attach the wires to the battery and asked the nurse for the screwdriver. Suddenly, from underneath the swathes of green sterile towels came a voice: 'A screwdriver! I'm lying here with my heart opened up and the doctor is asking for a screwdriver!' After the pacemaker had been stitched in, the doctor wanted a special magnet to test the pacemaker. Again: 'A magnet! First a screwdriver, now a magnet – what is this, an ironmonger store?'

Once the position of the wire or wires is satisfactory they are sewn in to stop them moving. A small space is then created between the chest muscles and the skin for the pacemaker battery. This procedure can sometimes cause discomfort for a short time. The wire or wires are then connected up to the battery and the wound is sewn up. Modern pacemakers are hardly noticeable under the skin once the scar has healed.

Regular pacemaker checks are carried out in special

pacemaker clinics, usually just before the patient goes home then a month afterwards and then at six-monthly or yearly intervals.

Living with a pacemaker

As with all procedures, complications can occur, the most common being when one of the wires becomes displaced, in which case it has to be repositioned. Some extraordinary things can happen if a wire moves. It can stimulate the breathing muscle or diaphragms, so the patient may come in saying: 'Doctor, hic, should I hic, be doing this hic, hic all the hic, time, hic?', which may be distressing for the patient but is amusing for everyone else!

Sometimes the pacemaker becomes infected. After all, it is a foreign body and, although it cannot be rejected like a transplanted organ, unless great care is taken infection can be introduced. This can cause a nasty illness and may even necessitate the pacemaker being removed. Nowadays most cardiologists give patients antibiotics immediately before and for a few days after the pacemaker is fitted to help prevent infections.

Once the procedure is finished and everything is healed we tell patients to forget about their pacemakers and to lead a normal life. Obviously certain precautions have to be taken and I generally advise my pacemaker patients not to indulge in activities like free-fall parachuting or competitive karate, to avoid being marked by Vinnie Jones in a football match and not to take up American football! The only major precaution one really has to take is at metal-detecting sites such as airport security and similar electronic barriers. Many people with pacemakers travel abroad – all they have to do is tell the security people that they have a pacemaker and they will be checked manually.

THE HEART AS A HARE

Just as a slow heart rate can make people feel dizzy or faint, so a fast heart rate can also produce symptoms, the most common of which is palpitations – a word that strikes terror into most heart specialists. Every speciality has its nightmare: for neurologists it is headaches, for orthopaedic surgeons it is backache and for heart specialists it is palpitations. The reason for this is that although we receive many referrals, in the vast majority of cases we can't find anything wrong.

Palpitations is not a diagnosis or a disease, but a symptom where the patient notices their heart beating in a way they perceive as abnormal. Just as you can't die of a heart murmur, so you can't die of palpitations. The vast majority of patients with palpitations are only experiencing an exaggerated sensation of their own normal heartbeat, or perhaps a minor irregulary that has no significance.

Of course patients are not to know this and when people start noticing their heartbeat they start to worry. And what does worry do? Yes, you've guessed it, it makes the heart beat faster and causes palpitations. So there is a vicious circle whereby patients become 'tuned into Cardiac FM' and the more they worry, the more their heart palpitates and the more their heart palpitates the more they worry. Try to remember the last time a motorist cut you up by overtaking on the left-hand side or nearly knocked you off your bicycle, or the last time you sat an exam or attended an interview. Some people with claustrophobia get palpitations when they are travelling on the tube or in a lift; indeed any stress in life can cause an awareness of the heart beating. Drinking excessive amounts of stimulants such as coffee or alcohol can also cause the heart to pound faster and all these experiences cause a surge of a chemical called adrenaline, which makes the heart beat faster.

Palpitations are one of the classic symptoms of being madly in love.

Great composers have long recognised this. In Mozart's opera *Don Giovanni*, the country maiden Zerlina, whom the wicked Don tried to seduce, must convince her fiancé Masetto that she is still madly in love with him and has not been unfaithful. In one of the most beautiful arias in the opera Zerlina takes Masetto's hand and urges him to place it over her beating heart (lucky old Masetto). She then sings 'Senti lo battere – tocca me qua' which means 'feel it beating – touch me here'. What purer sign of true love could there be!

The discerning GP who takes a careful medical history can usually work out whether the palpitations are due to an increase in the heart rate and the force at which the heart beats as a normal response to everyday living or to a change in the rhythm of the heart. Sometimes a physical examination may reveal clues: for example, conditions like anaemia, where there is not enough blood, an over-active thyroid, a fever, or even pregnancy can all cause the heart to beat fast.

The key question is what is actually meant by palpitations. Does the heart seems to be pounding excessively? Does it race so fast that it is quite difficult to count the beats or does the heart feel as though it has missed or skipped a beat? It is also important know if the palpitations are regular.

Because most people have their symptoms intermittently it is unlikely the palpitations will obligingly occur at the time of examination. The patient's description of the experience can be very helpful, and a doctor may ask him or her to tap out the rhythm on the desk. If a fairly regular rhythm of around 100/110 beats a minute is tapped this would suggest a slightly fast, normal rhythm. This is known as a *sinus tachycardia*. If the patient taps out a rhythm of 170/200 beats a minute or more, this suggests a real change in the rhythm of the heart. If a chaotic, irregular rhythm is tapped out this suggests a disturbance to a contraction of the upper chambers (atria).

THE BUTTERFLY HEART

The upper chambers (atria) can go out of rhythm in several different ways. The two most common rhythm disorders are known as *atrial flutter* and *atrial fibrillation*. In flutter the atria beat very fast, at about 300 beats a minute. Flutter is a good word as it conjures up something akin to the rapid motion of a butterfly's wings. There is no way that an effective contraction and relaxation cycle could be achieved 300 times a minute or 5 times a second, so when the impulses travel down to the heart's 'railway junction' (the AV node) the AV node blocks out some of the impulses so they do not all get through to the ventricles. In this way, the AV node protects the pumping chambers (ventricles) from receiving too many messages to beat.

One of the most common types of flutter is when every other impulse gets through to make the heart contract and the alternate ones are blocked. This condition is called *atrial flutter with two to one block*. It is nearly always around 150 beats per minute, which is well within the ventricles' capability, and has a characteristic pattern on the ECG. It may cause symptoms of rapid palpitations, usually regular, and the patient may feel their whole body shaking and their neck and head pounding.

If you have a problem understanding the concept of how some of the impulses get through and some don't, imagine the AV node as an acrobatic goalkeeper. Shots are raining down at him from all angles (back to Chelsea again) and he is leaping about trying to prevent them going into the net. Every ball he saves or parries can be regarded as an impulse blocked and every one that passes him gets through to the ventricles.

When the filling chambers (atria) *fibrillate* they cease beating properly and generate haphazard, chaotic electrical impulses about 600 times a minute. They shiver and shake, bombarding our poor goalkeeper with 600 shots a minute! The more impulses that rain down the more will get through and because there are so many of them the ventricles will respond irregularly. The patient with atrial fibrillation may notice a heart rate that leaps around all over the place like a jumping bean. Because the heart beats so irregularly not all beats are the same strength. Some are weak and won't cause enough of a ripple to produce a pulse at the wrist, so counting the pulse may not give a true indication of how fast the heart is actually beating. To count the number of heartbeats accurately a doctor has to listen to the heart with a stethoscope. Atrial fibrillation also produces typical changes on the ECG which should be relatively easy for doctors to recognise.

Both atrial flutter and atrial fibrillation have a variety of causes. They can accompany an acute problem such as pneumonia and inflammation of the lining of the heart (pericarditis), especially after major heart surgery. They can occur in patients with high blood pressure, left inlet (mitral) valve problems or an over-active thyroid gland and sometimes they occur for no obvious reason.

These rhythm disturbances are not in themselves serious or life-threatening unless there is some accompanying structural heart defect. For example, if a patient has furred-up arteries and suddenly the heart is asked to beat at 150/160 beats a minute the arteries may not be able to deliver enough blood to make the heart cope with that demand and the patient could get anginal chest pains. If the mitral valve is very narrowed, or the pump of the heart is weak, the onset of rhythm disturbances like this may make the patient breathless or even make the lungs fill up with water, resulting in serious illness. However, this is not the rule.

Most people with flutter or fibrillation find their palpitations highly unpleasant. One fairly common cause of atrial fibrillation is over-indulgence of alcohol. I can truly sympathise with patients who suffer atrial fibrillation because I have experienced this myself. More years ago than I care to remember, as a junior hospital doctor, I passed my first set of specialist exams. The celebration in the doctor's mess turned into a Bacchanalian orgy and during the course of an evening I must have drunk a whole bottle of whisky. Spoiling myself further I smoked three or four large cigars and when I was finally helped back to my quarters in the early hours of the morning I was virtually comatose. I awoke some five hours later, not only with the totally deserved symptoms of blinding headache and sickness, but with the added burden of atrial fibrillation, my heart racing along at somewhere around 170 beats a minute. Like sea sickness, there were two stages to this illness: the first when I was afraid I was going to die and the second when I was afraid I was not! It was one of the most unpleasant experiences of my life and one which I never wish to repeat. The thought of the various treatments which might be meted out to me made me too terrified to call for help, assuming I could have found the telephone! Fortunately several hours later my heart returned to a normal rhythm on its own. Never again!

Treating irregular heart rhythms

The treatment for flutter and fibrillation depends on how ill the patient is and how long they have had the condition. Sometimes, surprisingly, patients are found to have these abnormal rhythms at a routine examination for something else such as a pre-employment medical. They may have noticed nothing. The reason for mentioning this is that we may have no idea how long the patient has had this abnormal rhythm and must decide whether to try to restore a normal rhythm, or to try to slow down the heart rate by giving drugs which block even more of the impulses by, if you like, adding a second goalkeeper.

Many factors go into this decision-making process. If atrial flutter complicates a bout of pneumonia or if the patient has an over-active thyroid we must treat the underlying condition first and only try to restore the rhythm to normal when the patient is better. If the patient has only recently started suffering from fibrillation and the underlying cause is cured we would give a short-acting general anaesthetic and switch the heart back to the normal rhythm by giving an electric shock across the chest, using the same machine (a defibrillator) used in cardiac arrests. Sometimes we would postpone this treatment until the patient's blood has been thinned with warfarin for a month. The reason for giving warfarin is discussed below.

If the patient has a chronic underlying problem such as an abnormal left inlet (mitral) valve it is unlikely the heart will ever go back to a normal rhythm and treatment will be geared towards keeping the heart rate under control with various medications. There are millions of people walking around the planet with fluttering or fibrillating hearts who are quite well and living normal lives.

More difficult to deal with are those patients whose hearts keep flipping in and out of a normal rhythm, sometimes beating normally and sometimes fluttering or fibrillating. This is called *paroxysmal*, which is jargon for intermittent flutter or fibrillation. The change in rhythm can be particularly distressing for patients and we would therefore attempt to give drugs which try to prevent the filling chambers (atria) going out of normal rhythm. These drugs are known broadly as 'atrial stabilising agents' and they work with varying degrees of success. The choice of drug depends upon several other factors such as whether the patient has a normal or abnormal pumping function, the age of the patient and whether there are any other underlying conditions. This is because some of these drugs have side-effects.

In some cases we can't stop the heart going in and out of flutter or fibrillation and if the symptoms are very distressing drastic action has to be taken. Radio frequency waves can be used to destroy part of the electrical wiring system, so severing the connection between the filling and pumping chambers. This is done by putting a special wire into the right-side pumping chamber (ventricle) through the vein in the groin and 'microwaving' part of the electrical system. The jargon for this is *radio-frequency ablation*. This procedure doesn't stop the filling chambers (atria) doing what they want but it stops the patient knowing about it because the ventricles will no longer receive any messages. The downside is that if we destroy the mechanism by which the heart receives messages, the heart must be supported by an artificial pacemaker. Some patients find this acceptable because their troublesome symptoms vanish.

In the majority of cases the only major complication, particularly from fibrillation, is that blood clots can form inside the atria, probably because the blood doesn't move around. These clots may break off, travel through the circulation and get stuck somewhere else. The most dangerous place for a clot to go is into the brain, where it can cause a stroke, so measures must be taken to prevent strokes in people with fibrillation. In some cases this involves using aspirin but a true blood-thinning drug called warfarin has been shown to be more effective. I am often asked if warfarin is rat poison – it is! However, the idea is not to poison patients but to give them sufficient warfarin to thin the blood enough to make strokes very unlikely.

Patients on warfarin need regular blood tests to ensure that the drug is working effectively but not overthinning the blood. The administration of warfarin is usually controlled in special hospital clinics called *anticoagulant clinics*. It is a good idea if you are on warfarin to wear a bracelet or necklace which states that you are on the drug. It is quite possible to lead an entirely normal life while taking warfarin and, contrary to popular belief, alcohol is not forbidden. What we do ask though is that people drink a moderate but constant amount – the worst thing you can do when on warfarin is to binge drink, as this will really upset the apple cart and make your blood too thin. Also, certain other drugs, especially antibiotics, can temporarily interfere with the way warfarin thins your blood. The bottom line is that if you have fibrillation and you haven't been given advice on how to prevent strokes, please ask your doctor.

WARP FACTOR 8

The next group of fast heart rates (tachycardias) originates in the region of the AV node. These tachycardias are known as *nodal* or *junctional* because the AV node is the junction between the filling and pumping chambers. The mechanism of these rhythm disturbances is complicated and often involves an abnormal electrical pathway which evolved while the heart was growing in the developing baby.

Like all electrical pathways these abnormal ones are not visible to the naked eye and can even be difficult to see under a microscope. Many of us are walking around with pathways which we never use and which never cause us any problems. These pathways act as short circuits inside the heart. For example, if in addition to the normal electrical pathways there is a pathway which connects the filling chambers directly to the pumping chambers, with no 'junction box' in between, this produces a situation where there are two routes for the electricity to be conducted. Some of these pathways can only conduct one way but in certain circumstances the electrical signals can go down one pathway and back up the other one and whizz round and round in crazy circles like a demented Catherine wheel, producing rapid disturbances of the cardiac rhythm. There are several different pathways like this and sometimes they show up on an ECG as a bizarre pattern which inexperienced doctors may misinterpret as evidence of a past heart attack.

The best known of these strange abnormalities has the odd title *Wolff-Parkinson-White syndrome*, often known as *WPW*. (These weird names come from the people who described these abnormalities.) The full syndrome involves the abnormality on the ECG and a tendency to palpitation. Some people will just have the ECG abnormality without the palpitation. The conditions sound very high fallutin' and, as with the floppy mitral valve, some people get a lot of mileage out of them: 'I must take things easy, it's my Wolff-Parkinson-White syndrome, you know.'

On a more serious note, these abnormal electrical pathways can produce unpleasant palpitations due to rapid heart rates and cause characteristic patterns on the ECG.

Certain heart specialists look after electrical heart problems like this as their main interest, and treatment strategies have changed over the last few years. If the attacks occur infrequently, such as every twelve or eighteen months, it would obviously not be intelligent to put a patient on to daily medication because we would never be sure if the drug was working and drug treatment may be unnecessary. For people who suffer more frequent attacks drugs may be necessary and, as with flutter and fibrillation, there is a wide range for the heart specialist to try.

In the 1970s and 1980s, special cardiac pacemakers were developed which recognised when the heart went out of rhythm and put in paced beats which interfered with the Catherine wheel electrical pathway, breaking it and thus terminating the tachycardia. These pacemakers have largely been superseded by the microwaving technique I referred to earlier. In patients who have particularly disabling palpitations, or in younger patients who don't want to be committed to taking drugs for the rest of their lives, it is possible to map out fairly precisely the position of the short circuit and to 'microwave' it.

Mapping these pathways can be a long job and, like the x-rays dye test of the arteries, these procedures are usually done in special operating theatres dedicated to heart work. A few wires may be put into the heart, usually through a vein in the groin but sometimes also through a vein in the left arm. Using the electrical signals picked up from inside the heart, and by moving the wires around, one can locate the pathway and zap it. In expert hands this is an extremely effective technique and an abnormal electrical pathway is one of the few conditions we can totally cure. Not everyone with an abnormal electrical pathway requires this technique but it is a comforting option for those whose lives might otherwise be messed up by repeated hospital attendances.

Individuals who have these attacks infrequently may need to attend casualty departments where they will be given an injection of a medicine called *adenosine* which usually stops the tachycardia in its tracks.

Very occasionally conditions like WPW can cause very fast heart rates. These can lead the patient to black out and there are rare reports of people dying because the pumping chambers (ventricles) get bombarded with so many impulses through the abnormal pathway that they start to fibrillate, as they do sometimes after a heart attack. I must reiterate that this is very unusual.

THE SKIPPING HEART

The symptom of the heart missing a beat or an isolated thump is incredibly common. Although people may perceive the symptom as being a missed beat it is in fact an extra beat, often known as an *ectopic beat* or *extra systole.* Any of the heart's chambers is capable of putting in beats on its own at any time: beats arising from the filling chambers are called *atrial ectopics* and those from the pumping chambers *ventricular ectopics.* The heart may be beating away merrily when suddenly, for reasons which are not fully understood, an extra beat is put in.

This beat is sometimes felt as a fluttering or a bang in the chest but because the normal electrical sequence has been interrupted it takes a little while for the electrical circuitry to reset itself and these extra beats are therefore followed by a pause. This pause is known as a *compensatory pause* because the electrical system has to compensate to reset itself. This pause is often felt as a missed beat and some people become very disturbed by the sensation that their heart has stopped for a bit and may work themselves into a state. During this pause the heart is filling up and, as it has slightly longer to fill up than usual, the next beat after the pause may be slightly stronger than normal – a kind of super-beat. We thus have three components: the extra beat, the pause and the super-beat. Some people notice the extra beat, some notice the pause and some people feel a hefty kick with the super-beat.

Which chamber the extra beat originates from can be

determined from an ECG but, in any event, in healthy people these are nearly always totally benign and of no significance. They can, however, be worrying to the person experiencing them, especially as they classically occur when resting and not when rushing around during everyday activity. In some cases they are only noticeable when lying in bed at night.

There are few conditions which terrify people as much as the sensation of their heart stopping, with the associated fear that they are going to die. Needless to say this symptom generates a lot of referrals to outpatients. The condition is probably the cardiac equivalent of in-growing toenails – high in nuisance value but is low in seriousness! These symptoms can come in clusters: they will appear for a week or two, disappear for a few months and then come back. They are quite common at periods of stress or overwork or fatigue, during a cold or flu-like illness and sometimes they are made worse by coffee, tea or alcohol. Some people may only get three or four of these a day and find their lives devastated by them, whereas others may be getting thousands of extra beats during a day and not notice one of them.

Occasionally extra beats like this accompany something like a floppy heart valve (see Chapter 4) but even then they are unlikely to be dangerous. If the symptoms are devastating the beats can be suppressed with appropriate medication, but drugs like beta-blockers are usually ineffective and a specific rhythm-controlling drug has to be prescribed.

Sometimes these extra beats are picked up on a routine ECG. If we find no evidence of serious underlying heart disease we do our best not to treat these beats with medication because, as you will remember, all rhythm-controlling drugs have side-effects and we wish to avoid the treatment being worse than the illness! We therefore do our

131

best to encourage people not to focus their minds on their heartbeat because, as with other sorts of palpitation, the more you worry the more they are likely to occur.

OVERWORKED VENTRICLES

Most of the serious speeding offences originate in the pumping chambers and this is called *ventricular tachycardia* (*VT*). It is usually, though not always, associated with significant structural heart disease. Patients may experience not only palpitations but also dizziness and blackouts because during VT the heart's pumping mechanism may be ineffective and the blood pressure may fall. There are several different causes of VT but by far the most common is an enlarged and damaged left ventricle, which may be due to previously blocked arteries and heart attacks, muscle disease or damage to the muscle by valve disease that has been left too long. VT can occur in the early phase of a heart attack, even if the muscle is not severely damaged.

If VT occurs once a patient is on the coronary care unit it can usually be controlled by medication for a few days and then tends not to recur, unless the heart is seriously damaged. If a patient complains of rapid palpitations followed by severe dizziness or blackouts these symptoms must be taken very seriously. Sustained VT always requires treatment, even if the patient does not black out or feel dizzy.

Heart specialists spend a lot of time trying to find the cause of VT and patients nearly always end up having their arteries x-rayed and an echo scan, at the very least. Common causes include severe shortages of blood from the heart to the heart muscle, caused by furred-up arteries, a severely damaged pump of whatever cause, and HCM (see page 102). Sometimes however, we find these rhythm disturbances in people whose hearts look normal.

There is a whole variety of drugs available for treating these rhythm disturbances and the exact choice of drug will depend on how well the heart is pumping, whether the arteries are furred up, whether the rhythm disturbances are produced by exercise or occur at rest and whether the patient has any other conditions such as asthma.

Sometimes even powerful drugs may fail and we have to resort to other methods. In some cases it is possible to use the microwaving technique if we can find the exact source of the rhythm disturbance inside the ventricles. In the cases of people who have recurrent VT, particularly where it degenerates into fibrillation, we can now implant miniature versions of the machines which deliver electric shocks to restart the heart. These devices are called *automatic implantable cardiac defibrillators* or *AICDs*. When the heart goes out of rhythm they recognise it and deliver a small shock. The earlier versions of these were unsophisticated and bulky and their batteries easily depleted but the new models are much more reliable (although they still may require a lot of fine tuning). These AICDs have revolutionised our ability to treat life-threatening rhythm disturbances. However, they are very expensive and have done nothing to drive down the cost of medical care, but this treatment undoubtedly saves lives.

The only other treatment available for people with life-threatening rhythm disturbances is a heart transplant. Given that many of these patients have damaged pumps as well as rhythm disturbances this treatment is often appropriate and, of course, life saving.

So now you understand cardiac rhythms and how they can give you the blues!

7

WOMEN GET IT TOO

The popular image of a patient with furred-up coronary arteries is of a high-powered, highly stressed male executive who is overweight, may have high blood pressure, with at least two cigarettes in his mouth and one up each nostril. This image has been set in stone. More than a hundred years ago an eminent physician called William Osler described a coronary heart-diseased patient as: 'Not the delicate neurotic person ... but the robust, the vigorous in mind and body, the keen and ambitious man. The indicate of whose engine is always at full speed ahead.'

As this might suggest, most of the scientific studies on heart disease (including those which describe prevention, diagnosis and treatment) have been carried out exclusively on men. Heart disease is traditionally viewed as a male problem where the role of women is relegated to that of helping her poor husband to stop smoking, cooking him a healthy, low-cholesterol diet or helping him to cope with stress. After all, how many Health Education advertisements or posters for publicity campaigns have shown a woman clutching her chest or being rushed into hospital with a heart attack? Similarly, most of the advertisements in medical journals for drugs for heart disease show images of men.

Given this, women may feel that heart disease does not concern them and therefore may fail to recognise dangerous symptoms in themselves which they might spot in their husbands or fathers.

Statistics, however, tell a different story. Admittedly, the death rate from coronary heart disease in women is lower than in men of the same age, and never quite catches up with that of men (although the difference decreases with age). On the whole, the disease occurs between ten and fifteen years later in women than in men.

Despite the fact that most deaths from heart disease occur in older age groups, a staggering statistic is that coronary artery disease is also the single most common cause of death in younger women. In 1992 over 5800 women under the age of 65 died from furred-up coronary arteries in the UK, compared with 5690 deaths from breast cancer and 900 deaths from cancer of the cervix in the same age group. Yet publicity campaigns for early screening for breast cancer and justifiable outcries about misread cervical smears have been far noisier than campaigns addressing the real problem of heart disease in women. Yes, the female heart has had a raw deal!

I am afraid that many doctors seem also to have been brainwashed into regarding heart disease as a largely male illness. Well Women Clinics, for example, have traditionally focused on breast and cervical cancer, but the above statistics show that there really is no case for leaving out screening for heart disease in such clinics.

RISK FACTORS

To help understand heart disease in women, we should look at the way that the different risk factors outlined in Chapter 2 affect the sexes differently.

Smoking

One of the most worrying factors which has implications

for future generations of women (as well as their medical advisers!) is that the difference in smoking levels between adult females and males has virtually disappeared – in fact, girls are now more likely to smoke than boys. Peer pressure among teenage girls to start smoking seems enormously high. Although individual cases of young people dying suddenly from the use of substances such as Ecstasy make the national headlines for a few days – and quite rightly so – the insidious threat to women's health from the rise in cigarette smoking is likely to take a much greater toll than illegal drugs. Women who smoke more than forty cigarettes a day have a twenty times greater risk of furring-up their coronary arteries than non-smokers.

I spend ages reading the riot act to patients with heart disease who have been smokers, and my impression is that women are less likely to give up smoking than men, in spite of good intentions – I feel as if I am banging my head against a brick wall. Remember that by the time you have actually had a heart attack, the effect of stopping smoking will be much less than if you had never started in the first place or if you had given up at a much earlier age.

At the risk of sounding autocratic (who – me?), there are things I believe we all can and should be doing about the situation. Not only does the medical profession have a duty to keep hammering home the message on smoking but there is also a need to foster a change of attitude to smoking among teenagers. The media could help by stopping creating images in women's magazines and on stage and screen that turn women who smoke into positive role models. It may be that should we ever have a government enlightened (or brave?) enough to support a complete ban on cigarette advertising, the number of young people who take up smoking would diminish.

Diet and obesity

Generally speaking, British women eat a worse diet than men do. We unravelled earlier the jargon surrounding the use of words like 'saturated', 'polyunsaturated' and 'mono-unsaturated' fatty acids. If you skipped the chapter or have forgotten the information, I promise not to be offended (although you might wish to go back and re-read it)! Anyway, women appear to take more saturated or 'bad' fatty acids in their diet as a percentage of their food than men do. In addition, women's fibre intake is lower than men's and fibre, which is usually provided by vegetables and fruit, is beneficial in removing cholesterol from the body. Fruit and vegetables also contain helpful chemicals known as anti-oxidants which may stop arteries furring up.

In 1990 the World Health Organisation recommended that all adults should eat at least five portions of fruit and vegetables a day. Some groups in the UK consume less than half that. Recent information suggests that although women are increasing their fruit consumption, their vegetable consumption is still very low.

In Scotland, which has the highest risk of furring-up coronary arteries in Britain, a surprising number of women do not eat any fresh fruit or green vegetables. Low fruit and vegetable consumption could be an important contributor to the high rates of heart disease among women in Britain. I can still hear the shrill orders barked at me by nanny when I was a child to 'eat your greens'. Good advice!

Obesity contributes to the development of furred-up arteries in women and even mild and moderately over-weight women have an increased risk. The difficulty is that many of the effects of obesity may be related to allied factors, such as diabetes, high blood pressure or high cholesterol levels. To get this in perspective, however, a thin, smoking woman is at much greater risk from heart disease than a fat non-smoker. That is why, from the medical point of view, doctors do not mind when a patient puts on a stone when they stop smoking. But, of course, being the narrow-minded sexist individuals that we are, we may not recognise that an extra stone for a woman has other social and aesthetic results. While a man does not necessarily feel less sexy or less attractive if he gains a stone in weight, weight gain in a woman may affect her ego, her feel-good factor, her ability to wear favourite outfits and her perception of her physical attraction to her partner.

This may be one of the reasons that women may be more reluctant to give up smoking than men, and teenage girls and young women may see smoking as an effective means of weight control! Society promotes thinness as a feminine ideal. Just look at the fashion models on the catwalk. Not everybody adores the Kate Moss look, however, and some would regard the demoiselles of Renoir as more feminine. The Lucian Freud look is probably over the top!

Cholesterol

In both sexes the risk of furred-up arteries increases as the level of cholesterol in the blood rises, but women seem to tolerate a high choesterol level better than than men. One research study, for example, showed that even when the level of cholesterol was very high, i.e. greater than 7.6, only 10 women per 1000 aged between 35 and 64 years would get diseased arteries, compared to 26 men per 1000 in the same age group. The menopause causes cholesterol in the blood to rise. However, even after the menopause the effect of high cholesterol is not as dramatic as it is in men.

As further evidence of 'discrimination' against women, the clinical trials looking at the effect of lowering cholesterol on heart attack rates have always been confined to men. In late 1995, a Scottish cholesterol study showed that a drug which lowered cholesterol reduced the amount of heart attacks in men. But where, oh where, are the studies on women? The limited information there is suggests that when a woman has coronary artery disease, lowering cholesterol has a beneficial effect, just as it does in men. To explore this further, however, we need to have statistics from mass cholesterol testing in women. The chances of anyone conducting a large clinical trial of cholesterol-lowering drugs in a solely female population, however, are about as high as my chances of winning the National Lottery!

There is also the question of the reliability of plugging information from a Scottish male population into a geographically different population of females, especially as there are large regional differences in the incidence of heart attacks around the country. A publication from the Department of Health in 1993 reported the death rates in women under 65 as 11.5 per 100,000 in Cambridge, compared to 48 per 100,000 in Rochdale!

Here I must correct some popular misconceptions. The first is that high cholesterol inevitably implies increased risk of a heart attack (it does not) and the second is that high cholesterol means some genetic abnormality (it does not). Another misconception is that most people with high cholesterol levels in the UK are men. Believe it or not, the majority of individuals over 40 with high cholesterol levels in the UK are women. The effect of age on cholesterol levels is dramatic. But there is no point in measuring cholesterol for its own sake. It should be done in people who need dietary advice, as part of an overall risk assessment in heart disease, and to decide whether potential sufferers of heart disease need to take tablets to lower their cholesterol.

No studies have been carried out which prove that lowering the cholesterol in women who do not have any signs of heart disease is beneficial. Nevertheless, it is sensible to use cholesterol as one of a number of indications of increased risk, such as a bad family history, being a diabetic or having some evidence of arterial disease.

Diabetes

Diabetes increases the risk of furred-up arteries more in women than it does in men, with a diabetic woman having three times the risk of a non-diabetic woman.

The pill and HRT

Many people wonder whether or not the contraceptive pill causes heart attacks. This is largely because of periodic horror stories of thrombosis and strokes in women who have taken the pill. We know that the contraceptive pill can cause the blood pressure to go up as well as raising cholesterol levels. However, the risk of the pill contributing to heart attacks and blood clots elsewhere in the body is only a significant factor in women over 35 years of age, in smokers, or in women with high blood pressure. I would strongly discourage the use of the pill in either a smoker or a woman with high blood pressure.

The menopause seems to have an impact on the risk of developing furred-up arteries. Studies have shown that pre-menopausal women have a much lower incidence of heart disease than those of the same age who are menopausal. The most obvious question which arises from this is whether hormone replacement therapy or HRT affects heart disease. I wish there was a simple answer! The only way to be certain would be to do a huge clinical trial. This would involve taking a large group of women and dividing them into two groups exactly the same in terms of their cigarette smoking, weight and the incidence of diabetes. Half would then be given hormone replacement therapy and half would not. The two groups would need to be followed up for ten to twenty years to examine the incidence of arterial disease and heart attacks.

No such study has been done, although several studies have observed the effects of oestrogen replacement therapy over time. One large study looked at the effects of oestrogen replacement therapy on heart disease on 38,000 women over ten years. This suggested that heart disease in women on oestrogen replacement might be reduced. Scientifically, none of these studies actually proves anything, because you always need a control group *not* receiving treatment in order to compare the results accurately.

The currently prescribed hormone replacement therapy is the combined treatment using oestrogen and progesterone, but no one knows if this is as good, better or less good than oestrogen therapy alone. However, HRT is not without its drawbacks, the main one being the increased risk of breast cancer. As one would have to calculate whether the increased death rates due to breast cancer would wipe out the potential benefits of protection from heart disease, there would not seem to be any blanket 'Yes' or 'No' answer. A woman with a family riddled with heart disease but a low cancer risk might decide that the benefits outweigh the risks. Conversely, a woman with a very low risk of heart disease, say a non-smoker with normal cholesterol levels and blood pressure, but with two or three relatives who died from breast cancer, might take a different view. It will clearly take a long time to resolve this argument.

Exercise

Physical activity or exercise is often promoted as a way of

141

protecting the heart and arteries. There is some evidence that physical inactivity is an independent risk factor for heart disease, although much less important than smoking or high blood pressure, and that regular physical activity reduces the risk. Not surprisingly, studies leading to this conclusion have been carried out on men, and there is – yes, you've guessed it – very little scientific information about women.

There is plenty of evidence, unfortunately, that shows that inactivity is fairly rife in women. The 1990 National Fitness Survey graded levels of physical activity (0 to 9) needed to achieve a health benefit. It found that more than 90 per cent of women between 16 and 24 years old failed to reach the recommended target (level 5) for their age group. This level recommended vigorous activity, such as brisk hill walking, squash or aerobics that make you out of breath or sweaty, for periods of twenty minutes a time at least three times a week. Activity declines markedly with age – in the age range of 65–74, 40 per cent of women were scoring 0.

There are often social and cultural reasons why women exercise less than men; among some ethnic groups the idea of women exercising is not considered part of the culture. Many years ago I was asked by my boss to carry out a test involving bicycle exercise on a princess from the Middle East. She had never seen a bicycle, let alone ridden one, and after several vain attempts we all fell about laughing as she failed to master the art of pedalling! The majority of us use our legs more than eastern princesses, however, and there is some evidence that even walking for a mile a day is more energy-consuming than a half-hearted (no pun intended) attempt at aerobics once a week.

Exercise has beneficial effects on several factors which contribute towards heart disease. Regular exercise promotes weight loss, tends to raise the 'good' cholesterol in the blood, lower blood pressure and, of course, attention to physical fitness may stimulate smokers to stop. Physical activity should therefore be encouraged.

'Alternative' risk factors

Some odd and little known risk factors have been proposed. Recently published work from the USA examined three factors associated with ageing, namely baldness, greying of the hair and wrinkled skin. The earth-shattering conclusions from this work were that baldness correlated with heart attacks in men but not in women. The reason? There were too few bald women in the group! Surprise, surprise. The researchers claimed that there was a marked difference in baldness between men and women. Well, you live and learn. Grey hair was also impossible to evaluate in women, because up to 25 per cent of women dye their hair! Wait a minute, though, 43 per cent of women between the ages of 60 and 79 who wore wigs had a heart attack!

Another 'study' found that women who survived heart attacks had worse hearing than a similar group of women who did not have attacks. So, if you are a bald, deaf, wig-wearer from Rochdale, God help you! Honestly, with 'research' of this quality, we might as well suggest that the risk of a heart attack correlates with your star sign. Take heart, though, as skin wrinkling was only important in *men* under 55 years old!

A WOMAN'S PERCEPTION OF HER HEALTH

We have touched on women's attitudes to their own health in terms of smoking and diet, for example, and also looked at how the risk factors differ in women when compared to men. Of equal importance is the way that women with symptoms which might indicate heart disease are handled by their doctors. Changing attitudes have a part to play here. The fact that women have not been getting a fair crack of the whip has only recently been brought to light and, politically, heart disease among women is now a sensitive issue, or even a hot potato.

Perhaps because of the perception of heart attacks as a male disease, women tend to be less likely to recognise symptoms of heart disease when they have it, and take longer to seek help once they get symptoms. The 'indigestion syndrome' which I have been so rude about elsewhere is equally prevalent in women. Yet women will be much more stoical about chest pains or chest tightness than their male counterparts. A study reported in the *British Medical Journal* in 1994 found that women will put up with symptoms much longer and are more likely to call their GP than call for an ambulance, so delaying their admission to hopital. This delay in getting to hospital is bad news, because the administration of clot-buster drugs is more effective the earlier they are given (see page 58).

This delay reflects not only women's lack of awareness of the possibility of a heart attack but also an element of not wanting to make too much of a fuss. I recently had a case of a woman in her fifties who had deliberately concealed her symptoms from her husband for this very reason. Her symptoms steadily deteriorated and her GP referred her to a cardiac clinic. It was clear things were bad but even as she had her heart attack she hid her distress, and finally died. The ultimate tragedy of self-discrimination.

TESTS AND TREATMENT OF WOMEN

There is some evidence that women are more likely than men to have had previously unrecognised heart attacks.

This suggests that women may have experienced symptoms and ignored them, or perhaps had them dismissed by a doctor as being nothing to do with their heart. Studies have shown that doctors seem to be less likely to refer women for tests and treatment, again suggesting the possibility of a sex bias. These studies (mostly done in the USA) have also shown that even though their symptoms may be more disabling, women are less likely to be referred for the tests I describe in Chapter 9. The x-ray dye test (angiogram) which is used to map out the coronary arteries is used less frequently than in men, and in one study in London, less than a quarter of the patients who were referred for this test, having had heart pain diagnosed, were women. Another study from Northern Ireland found that women were five times less likely than men to undergo the dye test, even though a diagnosis of heart disease had been made.

As long ago as 1987 a study from the United States looked at what happened to men and women with abnormal radioactive scans (see Chapter 9). Abnormalities on these scans reflect areas of the heart muscle that are not getting enough blood on exercise. More often than not, these areas correlate with severe narrowings in the coronary arteries. Usually abnormal radioactive scans prompt the specialist to refer the patient on for the dye test of the arteries. In this study, sex differences were quite frightening. Abnormal scans were found in 31 per cent of women and 64 per cent of men. From the group studied, 40 per cent of men were referred for the dye test, compared to only 4 *per cent* of the women. After controlling for other variables, men were more than six times as likely to undergo the test. In spite of the results, the doctors were twice as likely to think that the women's symptoms were not due to heart pain.

Even in women who have undergone the dye test,

studies in the United States found that women subsequently had worse access to treatment than men, including balloon treatment or the by-pass operation (I'll explain these in Chapter 10). In 1993 research showed that among all patients with a diagnosis of heart pain, men were 50–60 per cent more likely than women to get either balloon treatment or a heart by-pass operation. No matter how many studies one looks at, women always come out worse off.

The National Forum for Coronary Heart Disease Prevention has tried to look at the reasons why women get such short shrift. These include the following:

Heart disease may be worse in men.

There is no evidence to support this. Women tend to seek medical advice later than men and have more advanced disease. Women are just as likely to die after a heart attack as men. The outlook for women with coronary narrowings is just as bad as it is in men.

Women with cardiac symptoms may be less likely to have coronary disease.

Heart pain in women may be associated with normal coronary arteries, as is described below. Many doctors, therefore, believe that nearly all women with heart pain are likely to have normal arteries and will come to no harm. This may be true in younger women but is not true in older age groups and the difference in the use of tests applies even among women who have had proven heart attacks.

Doctors may not think that tests are as accurate in women.

As discussed in Chapter 9, the treadmill test may throw up results which tell us disease is present when, in fact, it is not. This is particularly the case with women. Radioactive scans, although not perfect, largely overcome this problem.

Doctors may think that treatment is less effective in women.

Some studies in the 1970s and 1980s found that surgery had a less favourable outcome in women and women had less relief from symptoms. Improvements in balloon technology and surgical techniques have largely overcome this.

Women may be less willing to undergo surgery.

I do not believe that there is any evidence for this – in my own clinical practice I have not found women turn down the offer of investigation and treatment any more frequently than men.

Sex bias in the delivery of medical care.

The evidence that health professionals are less likely to refer women than men for treatment is convincing. A higher profile of coronary heart disease in men and the popular conception of this being a male disease may compromise the access of women to the same treatment. After all, one rarely hears of a woman keeling over from a heart attack in her forties.

To these explanations I would proffer one other:

Lack of communication.

Throughout this book we can see how easy it is for patient and doctor to talk at cross-purposes at what should be a simple medical interview. Another factor which can lead to a failure in communication is the barrier of language. We live in a multi-cultural, multi-ethnic society and some areas of the country have a high concentration of certain ethnic groups, among whom there may be a high prevalence of premature arterial disease. In some of these close-knit communities, knowledge of English is limited or even totally absent. My totally unscientific impression is that lack of English is more common in women from these communities than in men. A GP may find it difficult to obtain an accurate story and therefore refer the patient to hospital, taking the path of least resistance. Hopefully, the patient will attend an appointment with an English-speaking relative, but even then it can be just as difficult for the hospital doctor to unravel the symptoms, especially when questions are being asked and answered through a third party. A typical interview might go something like this:

DOCTOR:	Right, Your GP has told me that your mother has had some chest pain.
PATIENT'S DAUGHTER:	Yes, that is right.
DOCTOR:	Could you tell me what sort of pain it is?

Conversation between patient and daughter.

DAUGHTER:	It is a very bad pain.
DOCTOR:	Would you describe it as a sharp pain, a dull pain or a constricting tight pain?
DAUGHTER:	Sometimes it is sharp and sometimes it is just an ache.
DOCTOR:	Does the pain ever go down into her arm or into her jaw?

Conversation between patient and daughter.

DAUGHTER:	She does get pain in her arm.
DOCTOR:	Yes, but does the pain in her arm accompany the pain in her chest?

Conversation between patient and daughter.

DAUGHTER:	Sometimes yes and sometimes no.
DOCTOR:	Does the pain come on with physical exertion?
DAUGHTER:	My mother doesn't do very much physical

exertion.

DOCTOR: Well, can you tell me what would bring the pain on, for example housework or shopping?

DAUGHTER: She doesn't do any shopping and I do the housework.

DOCTOR: Well, you must be able to give me some idea of what brings the pain on!

Conversation between patient and daughter.

DAUGHTER: No, it is just a pain in her chest.

DOCTOR: Does she get short of breath with the pain?

DAUGHTER: She does get short of breath, yes.

DOCTOR: With the pain, or separately?

DAUGHTER: Separately, I think. (Conversation between patient and daughter.) Both.

DOCTOR: I presume your mum doesn't smoke or drink.

DAUGHTER: That is right.

DOCTOR: Has anyone in the family had heart disease?

DAUGHTER: Her father may have had a heart attack when he was about 50. And two uncles have also got heart problems.

At this stage, the doctor will examine the patient and have a look at a cardiogram which may be normal or show some subtle abnormalities which may not be specific for arterial disease. The doctor will have decided that the medical history is not going to be helpful, and may well be feeling frustrated that he or she cannot get through, directly, to the patient. There is a body language which doctors look out for when patients describe pain and this is absent when speaking through someone else.

It is even worse if the patient is not accompanied by an English-speaking relative. In such cases, the doctor will rely on the results of tests and will probably order an exercise test on a treadmill. If the woman can do a satisfactory treadmill test, the doctor would feel relaxed about reassuring the patient. However, like a bicycle, a treadmill is not a familiar instrument to many ethnic minorities, especially not to women, and they may find the test difficult to do. If they are unfit, they may become exhausted early in the test, developing fast heart rates at a low level of exercise. The test may therefore be hard to interpret.

If the test is abnormal, then the doctor has to make a decision about whether to put the patient on tablets and see whether or not the pain goes away; refer the patient for a radioactive scan or a dye test; or send the patient back to the GP saying that the pain is not likely to be due to the patient's heart.

All three of those scenarios are possible. In an ideal world there would be a perfect test which would discriminate between heart disease and every other disease with a 100 per cent accuracy. The nearest thing we have is the dye test, but resources do not allow us to carry this test out on everybody, and it is quite possible that our fictitious patient may not have received the right treatment, merely because of the difficulty in communicating on a one-to-one basis.

Another factor which militates against women from certain ethnic groups is the 'subsidiary' role which women occupy in these societies culturally. If women are not allowed or encouraged to keep hospital appointments because it is not convenient for their husbands, brothers etc to let them go or to accompany them, there is little the doctor can do.

'SYNDROME X' (HEART PAIN WITH NORMAL ARTERIES)

This is just about one of the most difficult conditions for a heart specialist to get to grips with. There is a large group of people, sometimes referred to outpatients or sometimes even admitted to hospital as an emergency, with symptoms that sound like classical heart pain. These patients are usually women in their forties, fifties or sixties who describe a heavy feeling, or tightness in their chest, often with shortness of breath. Sometimes they get this on exertion or sometimes when at rest, with pain also felt in the arm. Some of these patients will have one or two risk factors, such as being smokers, but many will have no identifiable risk factors at all.

There is usually nothing to find in such patients, so the doctor goes ahead and organises a walking test on a treadmill. Some of the patients will experience their symptoms on the treadmill, some will get no symptoms but have an abnormal heartbeat trace and some will have both symptoms and an abnormal trace. Some of the patients who have had symptoms while at rest will end up in hospital on a drip. They may have to wait in hospital for two to three weeks while a bed becomes available at a centre that can carry out a dye test.

Once this test has been carried out, a large proportion of these women will be shown to have no identifiable narrowings in their coronary arteries. What we are left with is a patient with symptoms suggestive of heart pain, an abnormal walking test and normal arteries. A minority of these patients' symptoms will disappear with reassurance, but over 70 per cent will continue to get symptoms in spite of knowing their arteries are normal. For want of a better descriptor, this strange condition has been called *Syndrome X*.

As you can imagine, when we resort to having to call something 'Syndrome X' it means we know very little about it, a bit like Planet X! It is far more common in women than men, and may respond to certain anti-anginal tablets, but the response is variable. The condition is often cyclical and may have come with clusters of attacks of chest pain for a month or two, then disappear or wane for a few months before returning with a vengeance. Sometimes, even when patients have been reassured that there is nothing wrong with their arteries, they still turn up in casualty with an attack of pain because they are frightened.

This condition is frustrating for patient and doctor alike. It is frustrating for the patient because the doctor has failed to identify a cause for what are undoubtedly troubling symptoms, and it is frustrating for the doctor, who is powerless to treat a condition whose cause is so poorly understood.

Quite a lot of research has focused on the behaviour of arteries in Syndrome X and people have put forward all sorts of possible causes. These range from a theory that the capillaries (the tiny blood vessels that give up oxygen to the tissues) have a problem with oxygen delivery, or that there may be a disease of the heart muscle that makes it use oxygen inadequately. In the early 1970s, it used to be thought that the condition was entirely psychological and that the only label that could be attached to these women was 'bonkers'! I am glad to say that the profession has become somewhat more enlightened; the fact that Syndrome X occurs so commonly in women compared to men, and particularly in the forties to sixties age group, suggests that there may be a hormonal influence due to changing oestrogen levels in the blood. Current research is focusing on this.

Some people have suggested that the pain may feel as if it comes from the heart when, in fact, it comes from the gullet. This suggests that more tests should be performed on the gullet. However, this is not usually a rewarding exercise.

No matter which approach a doctor takes, namely to try to convince the patient that the pain is not coming from the heart or to try to convince the patient that the pain may come from the heart but it is not serious, the symptoms remain. The outlook, however, is very good. Once you know that your arteries are normal, the chances of having a heart attack are virtually zero for the foreseeable future. However, the fact that we, as heart specialists, have failed to identify what the pain is does not make the pain any less real. Sometimes relief can be obtained by using a spray under the tongue (GTN is described in Chapter 10).

Cardiologists can expect to see more and more heart disease in women as the population of the United Kingdom ages, and the proportion of women in that population increases. Health professionals at all levels need to be aware of the risk of heart disease in women and to make sure that the obvious bias against women is corrected. It is equally important that parents, teachers, public health officials and doctors do all in their power to eliminate the risk factors that turn today's healthy teenage girls into tomorrow's unwelcome heart statistics.

8

DIPPING YOUR TOE INTO THE WATER
YOUR FIRST VISIT TO THE GP

Nicole: Papa!
Papa: Nicole!
This brief exchange in the well-known advertisement manages to convey perfectly the message that the car manufacturer intends. The interview between doctor and patient is a more complex process.

The success of a consultation depends on the experience of the doctor, his or her attitude towards the patient and vice versa. Sometimes doctors, whether they are GPs or specialists, have a 'bad day' when the last thing they want to do is to listen to other people's miseries. On such occasions doctors may convey an air of indifference or impatience – particularly if they are overworked, have been called out in the night or are suffering from a hangover! There is nothing magic about a doctor's constitution. He or she is subject to the same changes of mood and reactions to stress as everyone else. In the league tables of respect medics sit near the top, ahead of estate agents and politicians. But there is no guarantee that all doctors will be good at their jobs. There are good and bad doctors just as there are good and bad judges, lawyers and MPs.

Unless you are taken into hospital as an emergency via a 999 call it is likely that your first point of contact will be your GP. It can be a lottery as to whether you will have a sympathetic and conscientious GP or one who acts as a traffic policeman, directing patients with any symptom straight towards the appropriate specialist. Hospital doctors come to know pretty quickly who are the good and bad GPs in their area but there is little information available to the public about the quality of GPs. This is a fact of life and unless the politicians extend their league tables into general practice it is one we will have to live with.

Even if we had league tables it would be difficult to judge the quality of a GP. Should a GP risk giving a patient a course of treatment first, before referring to a specialist, or should an immediate referral be made in order to take no chances? In the first case the GP could either be praised for avoiding unnecessary referrals, or condemned for overstepping his or her area of expertise. In the latter case the GP might either be criticised for being no more than a clerical worker sending out letters of referral or praised for getting a patient into the hands of an expert as soon as possible.

Your GP practises family medicine and in a morning surgery may see patients with in-growing toenails, varicose veins, headaches, skin rashes, temperatures, gynaecological complaints and psychosocial problems. Not surprisingly your GP cannot be an expert in all these fields. In the limited time available a family doctor has to work out who needs reassurance and a pat on the back, who needs antibiotics, and who among this medical minestrone, requires referral to hospital.

TALKING TO YOUR GP

Although patients may feel guilty about wasting their doctor's time over problems they perceive as trivial I have lost count of the number of significant illnesses have been discovered from so-called minor complaints. People often feel intimidated in the presence of their doctor and for some people the doctor's surgery is reminiscent of the headmaster's study at school.

Even the process of making an appointment can be intimidating. Many GPs are protected by ferocious receptionists who ensure that in no circumstances are patients allowed to speak to the doctor on the telephone. These receptionists protect their GP as a lioness protects her cubs. If it is any consolation I also have problems trying to get through to GPs. I may have to repeat five or six times that I am a consultant, unbelievably important, and yes I do know the doctor is with a patient and no I can't phone back in half an hour and yes I am in fact returning a call that the GP made to me.

Once you have been granted your audience for three weeks next Tuesday, how should you approach your appointment? Remember that it is not the doctor's job to smile benignly at you over half-moon glasses but to reassure you when necessary, to investigate suspicious symptoms appropriately and never to intimidate or patronise. When doctors take a patient's medical history they rely on being given an accurate account of the symptoms and will often ask leading questions. Just as some doctors are better listeners than others, so some patients are better than others at giving an account of their symptoms.

The doctor is there to help you and if you have a GP who is not prepared to give you the time necessary, for goodness sake don't make things worse by being apologetic, as in the following consultation.

DOCTOR: It's Mr Johnston, isn't it?

PATIENT: Sorry to bother you, doctor, I know how busy you are.

DOCTOR: What can I do for you?

PATIENT: I've got this indigestion, you see, in my chest – I didn't really want to come but my wife ...

DOCTOR: How long have you had it?

PATIENT: Oh, on and off for the last couple of weeks.

DOCTOR: Yes, I see. What does it feel like?

PATIENT: Well, it's like indigestion.

DOCTOR: Does it come on after a meal and do you bring up wind?

PATIENT: I have wind sometimes and I have had it after a meal especially ...

DOCTOR: Do you smoke and drink?

PATIENT: I stopped smoking last year and I don't drink in the week but ...

DOCTOR: Well, you've probably got an ulcer or a hiatus hernia. Slip your shirt off and I'll have a look at you.

The doctor will probably give the patient a cursory examination and prescribe some antacid medication – usually that dreaded white chalky liquid or some tablets.

Before my friends and colleagues ring me up in outrage, let me say that this is not typical of how most doctors behave, although some do. Also, such an inadequate interview is by no means confined to the GP – I have seen and heard brief and inadequate consultations like this in casualty departments and in outpatients.

The interview started on the wrong foot and remained there. The patient was apologetic for turning up in the first place and allowed his answers to be continuously interrupted. The doctor accepted the patient's assumption that the diagnosis was indigestion. You will know by now that I am not fond of the word indigestion! You can help by not assigning or assuming a self-diagnosis but by giving clear descriptions of your symptoms. Even if patients do label their own symptoms the doctor should do some simple detective work to delve a bit deeper. This is how the interview should have been conducted:

DOCTOR: It's Mr Johnston, isn't it?

PATIENT: Good morning, doctor, thank you for seeing me.

DOCTOR: How can I help you?

PATIENT: Well, I've got this indigestion in my chest.

DOCTOR: Let's not use words like indigestion, because that assumes we know what is wrong with you. Can you describe exactly what you're feeling? Is it really a pain?

PATIENT: It's not really a pain doctor – it's ... well ... like indigestion.

DOCTOR: Would you say it was a sharp, stabbing sensation or a hot burning feeling, or is it more like a tight band around your chest?

PATIENT: Yes, that's it – it's exactly like a tight band.

DOCTOR: Does it feel as though there's someone standing on your chest?

PATIENT: Yes, I suppose it does, except more like an elephant standing on my chest than a person.

DOCTOR: Can you tell me what brings this on?

PATIENT: It seems to come on when I walk to the station in the morning or when I run up the stairs.

DOCTOR: So, is there a consistent relationship between the tightness and doing something physical or exerting yourself?

PATIENT: Not always, no. Sometimes I can walk without getting any indigestion, sorry, this odd feeling.

DOCTOR: Is it more likely to happen if the weather's cold or if you walk after a meal?

PATIENT: Yes, I *do* get it if I do anything after a meal – that's why I put it down to indigestion. Also, I bring up wind – doesn't that mean it's indigestion?

DOCTOR: No, not necessarily. Heart pain can make you burp. Does it go anywhere else, such as down your arm or into your throat?

PATIENT: I have felt a heaviness in my right arm but I put that down to rheumatism. Anyway it can't be my heart can it – doesn't heart pain always go down the left arm?

DOCTOR: A lot of people think that but it isn't true. Now, are you a smoker?

PATIENT: About twenty a day but I've been trying to cut it down.

DOCTOR: What made you try to cut down?

PATIENT: Well, I was getting short of breath so I thought it was time to stop.

DOCTOR: Do you get short of breath when the tightness comes on?

PATIENT: I suppose when I think about it my breathing does feel a little bit uncomfortable when it hurts. You're right.

DOCTOR: Is there anyone in your family with a heart problem?

PATIENT: My wife's sister has a valve or something ...

DOCTOR: No, I mean a blood relative, such as a brother.

PATIENT: My father and one of his brothers had angina, I think.

DOCTOR: Have you ever had your blood cholesterol measured?

PATIENT: I think it was slightly high at a medical I had some years ago.

DOCTOR: OK, Mr Johnston, I'll examine you now, but I'm pretty sure you've got pain from the heart muscle, which is called angina.

Although this interview is longer than the first one, it only takes five minutes for the doctor to probe deeper into the nature of the pain. This conversation could just as well have taken place with a heart specialist as with a GP. Mr Johnston was helpful as he gave clear answers to specific questions.

As in American courtroom dramas, where attorneys are always being scolded by the presiding judge for leading the witness, some patients do allow themselves to be led down the wrong path. Try not to let this happen; above all, don't let the doctor put words into your mouth. On the other hand, if the doctor is using descriptions that would not immediately have sprung to your mind, such as 'tightness' or 'someone standing on your chest', but do fit your symptoms, then do say so.

A GP'S ASSESSMENT

Sometimes even the most careful questions will leave the

doctor uncertain as to whether the patient has heart pain or not. Although in Mr Johnston's case it is clear the symptoms are related to the heart, on other occasions it is obvious that the patient's pain is due to something else. For example, if someone comes in and complains of a sharp stabbing pain under the left nipple which is worse when they turn their head to the left, it is clearly not angina.

In between the obvious diagnoses lie a whole group of patients with what we call *atypical chest pain*, atypical meaning not typical of anything. Vague chest pains that may or may not have a consistent relation to exertion and which can come on after meals may be impossible to resolve without further tests. This is where the risk factor assessment comes in. A typical chest pain in a 25-year-old woman with no risk factors is extremely unlikely to be due to the heart. The same symptom in a 45-year-old man who smokes, has high blood pressure, high cholesterol and three brothers who have had proven heart attacks must obviously be treated differently (especially if the man is going grey, balding and has wrinkles! – see 'alternative' risk factors in Chapter 7). It would be inappropriate to refer the first patient to a heart specialist but wrong not to refer the second patient.

Other symptoms which might indicate heart disease are shortness of breath, palpitations, dizzy spells, blackouts and ankle swelling. Shortness of breath might indicate a whole host of heart conditions though not everybody who is short of breath will have a heart problem. It is the GP's job to try to make sense of the symptoms and to get some idea of which part of the body is causing the problem. Shortness of breath due to asthma, for example, might be accompanied by wheezing or whistling sounds from the lungs; pneumonia might be associated with a high temperature or shivering attacks. Specialists don't mind seeing patients who turn out not to have 'their disease' as long as the GP has done the basic groundwork – not just written a referral note to the first specialist who comes to mind.

OPEN ACCESS

GPs do have access to certain basic blood tests, to check for anaemia or thyroid problems for example. GPs can also organise chest x-rays and ECGs. Other tests available to GPs directly depend on the policy of the local hospital and specialists. For example, in some areas GPs may be able to arrange treadmill tests for patients with chest pain while in others patients need an outpatient appointment with a hospital doctor first, although not necessarily with a heart specialist.

There are pros and cons to giving GPs access to these basic tests and these depend largely on the quality of the practitioner. I would have no qualms about allowing a GP whose judgement I trusted to have access to treadmill testing for patients with definite stable angina or heart pain, or for patients with atypical chest pain. Open access like this would make life a lot easier for heart specialists whose clinics are heavily oversubscribed and where the wait to see a specialist can be months.

However, there is no such thing as a perfect test and the treadmill test must be interpreted with the aid of sound clinical judgement. Some heart specialists are afraid that a GP who receives a normal result from a treadmill test back on a patient with chest pain will assume that the patient does not have a heart problem and could deny that patient referral to a specialist. This attitude assumes that the GP will always get it wrong and the specialist will always get it right – which of course is not the case: there are many heart specialists who will not carry out further tests if the patient's treadmill test is normal or who may put the patient on tablets and send them back to their GP. I know of cases where the GP's persistence has led the specialist to take things further, even down to carrying out a dye test of the arteries, because the GP is convinced the patient has angina.

The greater worries about open access to treadmill testing are that patients who should not have a treadmill test might be sent for one. Patients at risk include those who have unstable angina or a narrowed aortic valve. In the former a treadmill test might provoke a full-blown heart attack and in the latter strenuous exercise could provoke unstable cardiac rhythms.

The only solution is either to accept the status quo, and permit only hospital doctors to refer people for exercise testing, or – and I think this preferable – to have a well-developed programme of continuing medical education for local practitioners. Such a programme would keep GPs up to date with new developments and would advise them about the sort of patients they should be referring for exercise testing or to a specialist.

One of the tasks of hospital consultants is to disseminate information about changing practice into the medical community. GP meetings are often held in the evenings and accompanied by supper. On these occasions a consultant gives a talk and lively discussion will hopefully follow. Some GPs have been known to slip in for the supper and then surreptitiously leave before the lecture!

Although open access treadmill testing may be contentious because of the small risk involved if patients are put inappropriately on the treadmill, the same argument cannot be applied to tests where there is no risk. The main danger of open access to safe tests is that the volume of patients will be too great for the system to cope with. However, if GPs were to refer the right patients for the correct tests it would shorten hospital outpatient waiting times and ensure that consultants see the patients they really need to see.

Heart murmurs and palpitations could be easily sorted out. I have described earlier that a heart murmur is a noise and palpitation is a symptom which may or may not be associated with abnormalities of the heart's rhythm. A GP who hears a heart murmur should be able to refer a patient directly for an echo scan which, as far as we know, is completely risk free. If the echo scan is normal the GP would be just as capable as a consultant of reassuring the patient. Similarly, in patients with palpitations, GPs should be allowed access to some of the monitoring technology available in hospitals (covered in more detail in Chapter 9). If a normal ECG is recorded during palpitations the GP, again, can reassure the patient. A huge number of people have palpitations which are the simple ectopics or extra beats – or just an awareness of their own heartbeat. If patients with benign palpitations were excluded from heart clinics the waiting lists would shorten drastically.

If a test shows something abnormal, the GP would be able to mention this in his letter to the specialist and the outpatient appointment could be prioritised accordingly. Without this back-up of test results a referral letter might simply say:

Dear Doctor,
This patient has a heart murmur. Please see and advise.

Such a letter would be marked 'routine appointment', which may mean several months of often unwarranted anxiety for the patient.

In order for this open access system to work properly there must be enough monitoring equipment and technicians available to analyse the results. Unfortunately, in many instances in the cash-starved NHS, this Utopian ideal is unrealistic simply because of a lack of resources. It is very difficult nowadays to recruit cardiac technicians to do these tests and in some hospitals the wait for an echo scan or a rhythm monitor may be weeks or months. At present, the time involved in waiting to see the specialist and to take a treadmill test, echo scan and rhythm monitor can add up to the best part of a year. If we could reduce the waiting time we would make progress.

It may well be that if GP fund-holding is here to stay, entrepreneurial GPs will seek arrangements outside their local NHS hospital which will enable them to have these tests carried out more quickly. Money talks and some GPs are resourceful enough to arrange for investigations to take place in the private sector, where, of course, there is no real waiting list. If the heart specialist is unable to organise cardiac tests in a reasonable time this is because of a lack of resources and the fact that, as with the heart muscle and its arteries, demand so often exceeds supply.

THE REFERRAL SYSTEM

Meanwhile, back in tthe real world, you are sitting in your doctor's surgery having complained of chest pains, shortness of breath or whatever. If your doctor thinks you are an emergency you will be advised to go straight to the local casualty department (assuming it hasn't been closed down) for possible admission.

An example of such a case might be someone who has had chest pain for 12–14 hours the day before, and has somehow managed to get an appointment with the doctor the next day. A good doctor who hears this will obviously not want to keep the patient waiting until a routine outpatient appointment is available. Depending upon the relationship that the GP has with the heart specialist the GP may telephone the specialist to discuss the patient's symptoms. I'm not suggesting for one minute that it is any easier for the GP to find a consultant on the telephone than the other way round but if the consultant isn't available there is usually a registrar or senior house officer to take the call. A good GP might phone the consultant's secretary to ask for an urgent outpatient appointment and most consultants will respond positively to such a phone call.

Assuming that the GP doesn't think the situation is an emergency but that a hospital appointment is required, he or she will then write a referral letter. The consultant's response will depend on two factors, the first being the quality of the referral letter and its legibility, the second the mechanism by which the referral letter gets into the specialist's hands.

The quality of referral letters varies enormously. The use of cereal packet tops (see page 54) is fortunately not widespread but whereas some GPs will have their referral letters neatly typed out and will include a detailed patient history, others will send letters which look as though a spider has gone for a swim in an inkwell and then crawled across the paper leaving an eight-legged trail of ink. The worst referral letters say things like:

Dear Sir
Big heart, second opinion please.
Yours etc.

or

Dear colleague,
Pain chest since long time. I think there might be something wrong with him. Hoping your kind attention.

When a specialist receives a batch of letters asking for

appointments and has to prioritise them into 'urgent', 'early' or 'routine' he or she can only respond to the information given. The examples above are not only of zero value in terms of information given but could have been written by someone with the medical knowledge of a duck-billed platypus. The worry is that a referral like this, assigned 'routine' from lack of information to the contrary, may be disadvantaging a patient who might really have something very wrong.

To be fair to GPs, many of them just do not have the infrastructure necessary to allow them to produce typed referral letters with sufficient information to help specialists prioritise the appointments. However, in other instances badly written referrals can just be due to laziness. The following referral letter is a true example of the sort doctors like to receive.

Dear Doctor

I hope I am not wasting your time with this problem but I am rather worried about this lady. She gives a three-week history of cramp across the central part of her chest associated with rapid palpitations which make her feel dizzy. This has happened on six or seven occasions in the last few weeks – always on exertion, never at rest.

She used to smoke twenty cigarettes a day until two years ago and both her parents had strokes. She had both ovaries removed seven years ago and has not been on HRT, which makes me even more concerned. I could not find anything remarkable on examination but I have done a cardiogram (copy enclosed) which looks as though she may have had a heart attack. She has two teenage children who are dependent on her. I would be very grateful if you could see her as soon as possible.

Yours sincerely

A referral like this will soften the hardest heart and the likelihood is that one would slot the patient into next week's appointments – even if it meant overbooking the clinic.

Referral letters may be sent by post or through a local delivery system. If you haven't heard from the hospital within a reasonable time, a phone call to the specialist's secretary might be a good idea. My secretaries will not be terribly pleased to read this because their phones ring constantly, but as this book is written for patients (and I am not the one answering the phones!), I feel I can give this advice.

Doctors seem to be busier now than they used to be and time is at a premium. It is more difficult to get to know patients and to spend time chatting with them because demands upon GPs and specialists have snowballed. I remember accompanying my father on his visits before I went to medical school and in those days there was always time for a chat and even a cup of tea. Sometimes this approach could be taken too far. My grandmother, who was a diabetic, had heart problems when she was in her seventies. Her GP was the nearest thing to a perfect human sphere – a large ball with glasses. He would enter the house and, before attending to my grandmother, would go to the fridge and help himself to a leg of chicken or make himself a round of salt beef sandwiches heavily laced with mustard. He would then tuck in, wipe his chin on a Pavarotti-style white handkerchief and only then attend to my grandmother. After the medical side was over he would loiter in the kitchen until he was finally offered the obligatory piece of cake. Only then would he leave. I doubt if the man ever had a meal in his own house.

IN AN EMERGENCY

If someone has heart attack symptoms (see Chapter 3)

during the night the best thing is to call 999 and get him or her straight to a casualty department. Even if the GP is called, the best advice will still be to dial 999, although some GPs will go to the patient's house to await the ambulance. However, many GPs use deputising services at night so it may not be your own GP with whom you find yourself dealing.

Night calls used to be an accepted part of general practice. My father, who was a GP, was used to being called out at night, particularly for home obstetrics. He must have functioned on auto-pilot because one weekend I was staying with my parents and had given the coronary unit their phone number. At two o'clock in the morning the phone rang in my parents' bedroom:

SISTER: Is that Dr Dymond?

MY FATHER: Yes.

SISTER: We have a patient here in complete heart
              block who needs a pacemaker.

My father washed, shaved, dressed in suit, shirt and tie – as he always did when called out – and set off. He had driven about three miles before he wondered where on earth he was going and why; he had totally forgotten that there was another Dr Dymond in the house! When he arrived home he shook me awake and all I can remember hearing is 'Bloody pacemaker ... Bart's ... get going.'

The role of the GP when dealing with a patient suffering a heart attack has been the subject of much debate. The GP can certainly administer pain killers and an aspirin. (The aspirin is not given for pain relief but because it makes the cells which cause blood clots less sticky and less likely to form larger clots and has been shown to be beneficial.) Should GPs also give clot-buster drugs in the patient's home, on the grounds that the earlier these drugs are given the more muscle is saved? Many GPs are reluctant to do this for very good reasons. First, they may not have an ECG machine available to confirm that a heart attack is taking place; secondly, they may not have all the equipment available to prepare the clot-buster drug for intravenous injection or to monitor the heart's rhythm while the drug is going in; thirdly, it can be difficult to administer these drugs in a confined space.

Generally, it is probably better that the ambulance whisks the patient off to casualty where the drugs can be given in the proper environment. There are exceptions, however. In rural areas where patients are far from a hospital the GP may well be equipped with all the paraphernalia needed to give the drugs before the ambulance arrives. In big cities however, this would probably only delay transport to hospital.

TRUSTING YOUR GP

It is important that you find a GP in whom you have confidence – not just someone to deal with your heart attack but someone you can talk to about any problems affecting you and your family. If you are not registered with a GP you certainly should be.

A GP is not there just to refer you on to a specialist or to write out prescriptions for tablets, so don't assume that you will need to see a specialist for every single problem. However, a patient with symptoms that might indicate a serious underlying heart condition should be assessed by a heart specialist. Most GPs will be only too pleased to refer you to a specialist when necessary, but if you recognise in yourself symptoms which I have set out in the previous chapters and your doctor is reluctant to refer you, do please exercise your rights and ask for a second opinion. Very few doctors will refuse this request.

Having said that, there are some doctors who, when asked for a second opinion will reply: 'You want a second opinion? Fine. Come and see me again tomorrow!' Few doctors, however, behave like the infamous GP in Scotland who, when asked if the patient could have a second opinion, would arrive the next day with his dog!

I hope – despite my moans – that I have managed to convey the importance of establishing a relationship with a GP in whom you can trust. Assuming this is the case, then please do not dismiss his or her advice. Even if you are under the care of a specialist, you will need the help of your GP. Your GP will in most cases know more about you than you think and will do a very good job in increasingly difficult circumstances.

9

UP TO YOUR NECK
YOUR VISIT TO THE SPECIALIST

Once you have overcome more obstacles than Indiana Jones and obtained an appointment with your GP you will find yourself waiting for the Ultimate Challenge – an appointment with the heart specialist (or as we are known nowadays, the cardiologist).

People are in awe of heart specialists as they assume we have total insight into this mysterious organ. Specialists know more about the heart than plastic surgeons or gynaecologists, but we don't know everything. Heart specialists of the mid-21st century will look back and laugh at what they will see as our primitive attempts to get to grips with heart disease.

In the previous chapter I mentioned that the appointment allocated to you will depend on the information gleaned by the specialist from the GP's referral letter. If you have to wait for what seems like an eternity for an appointment, please remember that the doctor can only prioritise according to the urgency perceived.

One lively lady breezed into my clinic and announced in a broad Glaswegian accent: 'Och, it's easier to get an audience with the Pope than to get to see you.' I was horrified to learn that my waiting list was longer than the Pope's.

Some cardiac clinics are busier than others and whether you manage to see the consultant will depend upon how many assistants he has in the clinic. The pressure to see as many patients as possible has increased and gone are the days when doctors could sit and chat with a patient for half an hour.

There are many reasons for the increased number of referrals to cardiologists. GPs may be more likely to refer patients with suspicious symptoms to a heart specialist than they used to be because they have been educated to do so and also because they may be frightened of missing something, with the prospect of litigation if they have. Also, the population is ageing and heart disease is becoming more common. In addition, with a move in many hospitals towards specialisation, general physicians, who see whatever cases come through their door, are becoming less common. Nowadays the pressure is on to see the appropriate '-ologist'. This is not always possible because, even in 1996, some districts in the UK do not have a properly trained heart specialist at their local hospital. I will discuss the implications of this in more detail when I come to access and availability of different treatments.

THE CONSULTANT AS GOD

There was a time when patients were almost afraid of specialists and would turn up to outpatients spick and span in their best clothes. Some patients would even have a haircut, and many patients would not speak unless spoken to and would call the consultant 'Sir'.

When I was a house officer the preparations made for the visit of the Great One on his twice-weekly ward rounds would include changing all the bed linen (nowadays you are lucky if you have any bed linen). As the consultant did his round the ward would be silent and the patients had to lie with their arms at their side. No visitors were allowed to be present, and you could have heard a pin drop.

At that time the consultants ran the hospitals while a

few administrators, usually called hospital secretaries, were very much the proletariat, whose job was to make the patrician consultants' lives comfortable. If a specialist was asked to see a patient on another ward the nursing staff would leap into action, find the appropriate notes and escort the consultant to the patient, remaining with him for the duration of the visit.

How things have changed! Consultants' ward rounds now take place among the general cacophony of normal ward activity. Visitors sit by the beds and consultants trip over newspaper trolleys and try to make themselves heard above the general caterwaul. Hospital administrators would probably prefer we were not there at all as we get in the way.

In our so-called classless society it is quite right that patients should not be deferential to doctors but the least they could do – bearing in mind that we have noses – is to wash. The Outpatient Feet Syndrome is one with which most doctors are familiar. Much publicity has been given to the Patient's Charter – a glossy brochure that sets out mission statements for the NHS – but there should also be a Health Service Worker's Charter. Some of the key points would be:

- All patients must have washed their feet and put on clean socks before coming to outpatients.
- Patients must turn up on time for their appointment.
- All patients will speak clearly and give a concise and accurate history, enabling the doctor to make a diagnosis easily.
- No patient will burp or break wind during their consultation.
- No patient will be inconsiderate enough to have a heart attack in the middle of the night and have the doctor get out of bed.
- All patients will have a kind and caring family, ready

to take the patient out of hospital when they are medically fit. (Ha Ha!)

PREPARING TO SEE THE CONSULTANT

Under the Patient's Charter you are supposed to be seen within half an hour of your appointment time. In practice this is not always possible. Clerical staff who run the clinic may be chasing missing notes, or results of tests which have not found their way back into the notes; patients themselves may be late arriving. Add to this all the other factors that can contribute to delays, such as having to talk to a patient by means of an interpreter or having a particularly sick patient to deal with, and you will see that it is not always possible to stick to scheduled times. Please be patient. The specialist has no wish to keep anyone waiting longer than necessary. Just imagine how you would feel if you had a particularly difficult problem: you would not want the specialist to say he was sorry but he couldn't spend more time with you because it was someone else's turn.

Before you go in try to have worked out a description of the symptoms troubling you. If you are on medicines please bring them with you or at the very least bring a list of your pills and their dosages. If you are able to give a concise history and an accurate description it is likely the specialist will have a good idea of what is wrong with you or at least be able to narrow it down to two or three conditions. It can be infuriating for a specialist to interview patients who are unable to focus on their symptoms or answer questions directly. For example,

PATIENT: Good morning, doctor. It's turned cold hasn't it.

175

DOCTOR: Yes, it has. Now, Mrs Brown, your GP has written to me saying that you've had some chest pain. Is that right?

PATIENT: Yes, doctor, although I haven't had it for a while.

DOCTOR: When did it first start?

PATIENT: Well, I went to visit my daughter, I think it was on the Friday – no, the Thursday – yes, the Thursday; she lives in Lincoln you know. Oh, she's got a lovely house with a pretty garden; it was the best thing they ever did to move up there. The air is better than down here and the shops are nice but ...

DOCTOR: Mrs Brown, can we get back to the pain in your chest? When did it first start?

PATIENT: Well, we'd just had lunch in town. I'd had one of those Italian pasta dishes with a beef sauce – no, wait a minute, my daughter had that and I had the chicken breast ...

DOCTOR: Mrs Brown, please tell me about the pain.

PATIENT: I'm coming to that, doctor. Anyway, after lunch we went shopping for presents for my grandchildren. I've got the two, you see, eleven and eight, and their birthdays are quite close and it seemed a good idea to kill two birds with one stone, as it were. Richard's the older one, he's crazy about football ...

DOCTOR: (with a deep sigh) Mrs Brown. If you don't actually tell me about the pain I really can't help you.

PATIENT: Sorry, doctor. Anyway, we were walking to the shops and the pain came on.

DOCTOR: Now, show me exactly where you felt the pain.

PATIENT: I can't, doctor. It was about half way down the High Street in Lincoln.

DOCTOR: No, no! I mean where in your chest?

PATIENT: Oh, I'm sorry, doctor. Well it was sort of ... I don't know ... here. (Mrs Brown points vaguely to an area on the left side of her chest.)

DOCTOR: OK. Now what sort of pain was it? I mean was it sharp and knife-like or was it a tight, heavy feeling?

PATIENT: Yes, just like that.

DOCTOR: Like what?

PATIENT: Like a knife and heavy.

DOCTOR: (now transforming into Basil Fawlty) Mrs Brown! It can't have been like a knife and heavy at the same time! Now please try to describe it.

PATIENT: Sorry, doctor. It was sort of a bad indigestion, you know. I put it down to the apple pie, being in a rush, you know and it came out between my shoulder blades. It was just like the pain I had when I hit my thumb with a hammer when I was trying to hang a picture at home. I suppose I shouldn't have been doing it, but left it for our Bert to do instead. Still, you can't just sit around waiting for other people to do odd jobs for you, can you?

At this stage there are two options open to the doctor. He or she can either have a nervous breakdown or change specialities and transform into Dr Hannibal Lecter and the patient will cease to be a problem!

It is clear that Mrs Brown would never be a good witness even if interviewed for a month. The consultant therefore has to rely on intuition and a few basic investigations but, as the story from the patient is of paramount importance, the process is unsatisfactory. This is the reality of medicine.

Some patients come in with predetermined ideas about what they will and will not undergo. A few months ago I saw a patient who had had a minor stroke. His GP had written a very good referral letter, asking me to exclude a cardiac cause such as a change of rhythm. Even before he sat down, and before I had a chance to introduce myself, the patient started off the interview by saying:

PATIENT: I won't take any chemicals.

ME: Good afternoon. I'm Doctor D——.

PATIENT: I don't want to know anything about my illness.

ME: Well, your doctor has referred you to me to see if your heart was responsible for your str——

PATIENT: Don't mention that word!

ME: What word?

PATIENT: That word. You know – the S word.

ME: OK, but there may have been a cardiac cause for the S word.

PATIENT: Even if there is I don't want to know about it. Please let me be an ostrich.

The patient answered my questions reluctantly and allowed me to examine him. He was willing to undergo a few basic investigations but, as I wrote to his doctor, 'Lord alone knows what we will do if the tests prove abnormal.' Of course it is a patient's absolute right to ignore illness and refuse treatment but it's a pity if some simple preventative medicine could cut out the risk of another S word.

Sometimes it is not the patient who has difficulty with the medical interview. Below is an interview which took place between a patient and a junior doctor from overseas who was training with us at Bart's. The doctor was attempting to ascertain whether the patient had any symptoms of excess fluid. As you will remember, one such symptom is ankle swelling.

DOCTOR: So tell me, how is your arnkle?

PATIENT: Do you know my uncle?

DOCTOR: No no! I want to know if your arnkle is swollen or not.

PATIENT: Well, he may be a bit overweight but I wouldn't say he was actually swollen. I'll tell him to come and see you.

This sort of misunderstanding probably happens more often that we would like to think. I once saw a Hungarian lady privately. She had her own brand of English which made it hard for me to get to grips with the interview, especially as she told me about her difficult family.

ME: Do you smoke?

MRS K: Oh, every blue moon, doctor.

ME: Is there a family history of heart disease?

MRS K: You wouldn't believe it, doctor. There are so

179

> many hearty dicks in my family, and my hus-
> band has blood pressure. He was a parmizan
> in the war, you see.

ME: Do you have children, and are they well?

MRS K: My children! My son breaks my heart. All his
girlfriends are bingos, and he wants to go off
hijacking around the world with one of them.
He hopes to settle in New York, but if you are
not rich there you are really in the gut. My
daughter is a crazy nutpot. She can't have
children easily so is on fertilisers. Mind you
she can make strudel with her eyes closed and
tied behind her back! I won't run around the
bush, doctor, I think my kids are the result of
my palpitations ... Anyway, doctor, let me
have your bill and I'll settle down with you!

Not only can communication difficulties be amusing but
also embarrassing. It is common for patients to be accompanied by their spouse or another relation so I didn't think
twice when, on one occasion, having called Mr Hoffman,
two people came into the consulting room. They sat down
opposite me and I began to talk to Mr Hoffman about his
illness. Mr Hoffman kept glancing to the lady on his left
while answering my questions and the lady sank lower
and lower into her chair, gazing at the floor.

When I had finished taking his history I asked Mr
Hoffman to go into the examination room; only then did I
take a good look at the lady and said rather sheepishly:
'You *are* together ... aren't you?'

'No! I'm very upset,' she said, trembling. 'I've got no
idea who that man is. Do you normally see two patients at
a time?'

It turned out that the lady had a surname not dissimilar
to Hoffman and she had thought she was being called in.

She was so intimidated by the situation that she failed to speak up. Even Mr Hoffman didn't say anything but, had I had my wits about me, I would have realised that they made an odd couple. I have since met her on several occasions and we still have a good laugh about it.

You meet all cross-sections of the population in outpatients. The proximity of Bart's to the Old Bailey means we have had our share of people involved in the legal process – from villains to High Court judges and even a couple of Law Lords – attending clinic. Your heart doesn't know if you are sitting on the bench wearing ermine or if you are standing in the dock.

One afternoon the truth of this was brought home to me when I had just finished seeing an eminent Legal Lord who was dressed in his NHS designer striped dressing gown. The next patient was a whale of a man, described as a mechanic. He was in his thirties and about to become a guest at one of Her Majesty's prisons for armed robbery. He was so huge and I wondered how anyone of such bulk could have hoped to make a quick getaway (well, obviously he didn't, hence the porridge).

ME: Good afternoon. I'm a heart specialist.

PATIENT: 'Allo, doc.

ME: Have a seat (have two seats). Now, what can I do for you?

PATIENT: It's me chest. I' 'urts and ah get art of breff.

I tried to take a medical history and we then came on to his habits:

ME: Do you smoke?

PATIENT: Yeah.

181

ME: How many?

PATIENT: Eye-ee.

ME: Eye-ee?

PATIENT: I smoke eye-ee fags.

ME: Oh, you mean eighty! What, about eighty a week?

PATIENT: Nah, eye-ee a day.

ME: And do you drink alcohol?

PATIENT: Yeah.

ME: (Here we go again.) How much?

PATIENT: Ore-ee.

ME: (now tuned in.) What? Ore-ee – I mean forty – pints a week?

PATIENT: Nah, ore-ee a day.

ME: !

I did some rough calculations on the blotting pad so thoughtfully provided by the NHS and worked out that between smoking and drinking eye-ee and ore-ee a day and the odd trip to the loo my patient's time was totally occupied. Maybe this would stop him from re-offending. While he lumbered into the examination room I found myself doodling the following rhyme on my NHS blotter:

I have now been referred a thirty-year-old mechanic,
He smokes eighty a day and drinks forty a night,
It's no wonder his hulk would dwarf the Titanic
And he's gasping for breath as his recounts his plight.

'I can't give em up,' he explains 'It's addiction,

To nicotine, alcohol, sarnies and snacks,
With the court case and stress of me recent conviction
I rely on me fags and me booze to relax!'

Is this worthwhile use of my clinical skill?
This patient's salvation is beyond medical sages.
The best advice I can give is to make out a will,
And not to start any novels with too many pages.

Ted Hughes's Poet Laureateship is safe for the moment!
This ditty was, I suppose, an expression of my helplessness
at trying to cope with what in the life assurance business
would be termed a 'severely substandard life'. My patient
had a collection of furred-up arteries, poisoned heart
muscle, soot-filled lungs and a pickled liver – all of which
had occurred as a result of self-inflicted abuse of commercially available chemicals. In cases like this I can do very
little except compose silly rhymes. My NHS blotter has
since been removed – all part of the cuts!

THOSE TESTS

To return to the serious business of outpatients, if you are
being seen for the first time, you will probably have an
ECG and possibly also a chest x-ray. The doctor should
explain to you what might be wrong and what tests you
will undergo. Most of the investigations will be as an outpatient and, depending on the results of these, you may be
reassured, put on medical treatment or offered the dye test
(angiogram) which will x-ray the inside your heart.

There is a logical process which determines the order in
which tests are performed. For example, if the doctor
thinks you have heart pain or is unsure about the nature of
your chest discomfort, a treadmill or walking test may be

ordered. If you are complaining of palpitations or if the
doctor wants to check the stability of the heart's rhythm,
some sort of monitoring test will be requested. If the doctor
wants to get an idea of the structure of your heart and the
thickness of its muscle an echo scan will be ordered.

When you leave outpatients you should be clear about
what tests you are going to have and why. If you are
alarmed or frightened about some of the tests, please don't
be afraid to express your anxieties. Nearly all the tests are
painless; only one or two outpatient tests involve having
an injection, although some of the inpatient tests involve a
little bit more.

Treadmill test (exercise electrocardiogram)

The exercise ECG is also known as an *exercise test*, a *stress
test* or a *treadmill test*. Its purpose is to make the heart work
harder so its performance can be examined under exercise
– pulse rate, blood pressure and the ECG trace are recorded
during exercise. Most tests are done on a walking treadmill, although in some places bicycles are used.

The first stage of the test usually involves a gentle walk
on a flat treadmill, i.e. without any gradient or incline.
Every few minutes the test is made slightly more difficult
by adjusting the speed of the treadmill and/or making it
tilt upwards slightly. Obviously the more work you can do
on the treadmill the more likely it is to provide good information for your doctor, so please don't cave in after thirty
seconds. It helps if you bring a tracksuit and a pair or tennis shoes or trainers as it is difficult to perform well on the
treadmill in stiletto heels! You should report any symptoms
such as chest tightness, shortness of breath or dizziness
during the test.

The test may be supervised by a doctor or a technician
but don't worry if there is not a doctor present as the

person doing the test will be trained to cope with any adverse consequences.

At some point in the test the person supervising may ask you to stop, even if you feel all right. There could be several reasons for this: you may have achieved the heart rate expected for your age, or the pattern of the ECG may have changed and given the answer we were looking for. Even if you have no symptoms, the rhythm of your heart may have changed or your blood pressure may have gone too high or too low. It is possible to have an abnormal treadmill test in the absence of any symptoms. It is usual to go on recording the pulse rate, the blood pressure and the ECG for some minutes after the exercise is terminated because changes which may indicate the heart is short of blood may not occur during exercise but may become apparent during recovery.

The test is not perfect. Sometimes it shows up abnormalities on the ECG trace when the heart is completely normal – these are called 'false positive' tests. The reverse is also true, in that sometimes the test will appear normal even though there is something wrong. The doctor must interpret the test in the light of all the clinical information.

You may have had a treadmill test as part of a health screen and if it showed any abnormality, another test, perhaps a radioactive scan of the heart or an x-ray dye test of the arteries, will be necessary.

It is difficult for doctors to ignore abnormalities which show up. Once an abnormal test has been recorded, you can't pretend you've never had the test in the first place but you have to go on down the road until the question mark is removed.

Not only is treadmill testing used to diagnose illness but it can also be used as a follow-up and to monitor possible change in a patient's condition. A patient with narrowed arteries may be asked to undergo treadmill tests at six-monthly or annual intervals. Patients may also be asked to undergo this test if they have had balloon treatment or a heart operation (see Chapter 10).

Echo scan

The echo scan simply involves having a probe moved over your chest in different directions to bounce sound ultrasound waves off your heart and build up a picture. The probe is covered with jelly to improve the signal.

There are many reasons for carrying out an echo scan and it can be repeated easily, being totally harmless. People with valve problems or artificial heart valves, suspected muscle problems or congenital heart disease, to name but a few, are studied in this way. You can watch the strange images appear on the screen but don't expect to understand them.

The only bit you may find alarming is when we use the Doppler technique. As I explained in Chapter 4, this is used to look at the blood flow across the heart valves. The test makes a loud whooshing noise in time with your heart beat and sounds like something out of a low-budget science fiction movie. The Doppler signal can be measured and even colour-coded so that we can see where abnormal blood flow is going. As mentioned in Chapter 4, we often now ask patients to swallow a small probe to scan the heart from the gullet. This isn't nearly as horrific as it sounds and helps to give accurate information, particularly in patients with artificial heart valves.

Radioactive heart scans

These are tests which heart specialists either love or hate. Not all hospitals are equipped to do these heart scans but, when done well, these tests can provide invaluable information.

Don't worry about being radioactive – you won't glow in the dark! The radioactivity decays naturally and some of it is passed out of the body through the kidneys.

There are two types of radioactive heart scan. The first produces a picture which represents the blood flow into the muscle of the heart; the second gives information on the heart's pumping function. The first is more widely practised than the second and uses a radioactive substance called thallium. The test itself is called a *thallium scan* (not a valium scan!).

In the same way that the resting ECG is not as much value as the exercise ECG, so a thallium scan is most often performed during stress or exercise. Usually, you will have a treadmill test and at the end of exercise a tiny amount of thallium is injected into a vein in the elbow. The thallium gets into the heart muscle in proportion to the blood flowing into the muscle down the coronary arteries. This means that in normal circumstances, where all of the heart muscle receives enough blood during exercise, the picture produced will show a uniform uptake of thallium. If part of the heart muscle doesn't get enough blood because one or more of the coronary arteries is narrowed or blocked, that piece of heart muscle will not take up thallium as well as the normal parts and the picture produced will show an abnormality. These pictures are usually produced in colour.

There will be another injection of thallium a short time after exercise, when the heart has returned to normal, and another set of pictures are produced which show the blood flow at rest. Just as the resting ECG can be compared with the exercise one, so the resting thallium scan can be compared with the one during exercise, and the areas of abnormality identified. All you have to do once the thallium is injected is to lie on the couch and doze while a special camera rotates around the chest, building up the picture. You will not feel anything but the radioactivity in your heart is detected by the camera and a picture built up with the aid of a computer. The quality of the picture depends upon the test being performed correctly. Many heart specialists are prejudiced against the technique because, if performed incorrectly, the final pictures end up looking a bit like a fried egg and are difficult to interpret.

One of the beauties of this technique is that we can mimic exercise by injecting certain drugs into the vein which have the same effect on blood flow into the heart as exercise. This makes it useful for people who can't exercise because they have arthritis or poor circulation in their legs. Also, a patient doesn't have to be physically fit to undergo one of these tests. During the injection of the drug you might feel a slight sense of flushing or pounding of your heart. The side-effects are usually minimal.

Thallium scanning is useful if a doctor is faced with an exercise ECG which is difficult to interpret or which he or she thinks may be 'false positive'. If the subsequent thallium scan is normal the patient can be reassured; if it is abnormal the doctor is likely to pursue further tests.

Newer radioactive agents have recently come on to the market, so if you have a scan like this don't be alarmed or surprised if thallium is not used and you have something with another name.

For the other radioactive test, which looks at the pumping function of the heart both at rest and during exercise, you might be asked to pedal on a bicycle while leaning against the camera. These tests don't take long and are no more traumatic than having a blood test.

Rhythm-monitoring techniques

Disorders of the heart's rhythm can cause palpitations, dizziness or blackouts. However, these electrical faults tend to be intermittent and rarely conveniently show themselves on an outpatient visit. Sometimes the specialist may have an idea of what is going on from the patient's medical history and from the ECG, but it is still important to try to document the rhythm change rather than to treat the condition blindly with a drug or a pacemaker.

If a patient complains of symptoms which occur nearly every day the doctor will arrange for what is called a *24-hour tape* or *Holter Monitor* (not, as one patient said, a Hitler Monitor!). Small electrodes are placed on the chest and wired up to a little box containing a slow-moving tape cassette, and every heartbeat for the whole 24 hours is recorded onto the tape. The patient wears this box, rather like a Walkman, around the waist. Patients should lead a normal life during the period of monitoring (except, of course, not going for a swim or jumping into the shower).

The patient will be given a diary and asked to note as accurately as possible when the symptoms occur so that when we play back the tape through a high-speed analyser we can correlate the symptoms with what the heart beat was doing when the symptoms came on. Sometimes we can detect abnormalities which guide us to treatment, even when symptoms are not present.

Patient diaries can often be entertaining, particularly at night! One female patient who had palpitations wrote a note at 10 pm:

'I am terribly sorry but I was just about to go to bed with someone for the first time and the tape machine would have got in the way so I took it off. I hope this all right.'

Another patient set out in lurid detail exactly what happened during a night of seemingly incessant sexual activity. My editor has prevented me from describing this activity but details can be obtained by writing to me enclosing a plain brown stamped addressed envelope!

Yet another patient, who among his many problems had difficulty performing sexually, found that being attached to a 24-hour tape revolutionised his sex life. The electrodes on his chest and the box strapped to his waist had obviously made him feel completely bionic and he wrote to me thanking me profusely for enabling him to perform properly for the first time in years. My one and only 24-hour-tape fetishist!

For patients who have their symptoms less frequently, monitoring one 24-hour period may be absolutely useless. In such cases it is better to work with a device which they can hold over their chest and record their ECG during an attack. These machines are easy to use and are called *cardiomemo* devices. They store the ECG signal in a computer-like memory and the trace can either be brought into hospital or transmitted down the telephone line to the hospital technicians. This can prove extremely useful in catching elusive symptoms. Obviously, someone who blacks out completely will be in no condition to hold a monitor at the crucial time, but a partner, spouse or other relation can be shown how to use it, provided they can keep a cool head.

A fairly recent test for people with unexplained blackouts is called a *tilt table test*. This is exactly as it sounds. The patient is strapped to a table which is titled at about 60 degrees and the heart rate and blood pressure monitored. Sometimes this produces a profound slowing of the heart rate and a drop in blood pressure. The trouble is that no one really knows what to do with the abnormal results. Even if we put in a pacemaker the patient may still go on getting symptoms, and various medicines can be tried.

The x-ray dye test (angiogram)

I have been using the colloquial term 'dye test' quite often when talking about x-raying the coronary arteries. This commonly used description is a little misleading, because the liquid we use is not a dye at all. It is colourless and contains iodine which shows up easily on x-rays. At no time does the blood change colour and the liquid is passed out in the urine without being noticeable.

This test involves coming into hospital. If you are on the waiting list the test will usually be done as a day case and you will come in the morning and go home in the evening. If you have been taken ill as an emergency you may well have been transferred from your local hospital into another hospital which can do the dye test, which is properly called an *angiogram*. The angiogram takes place in a special operating theatre called a *cardiac catheterisation laboratory* – often abbreviated to *cath lab*. It is also known as an *angiography theatre*, often shortened to *angio*.

When you go in don't be frightened by the array of equipment you see before you. There will be an x-ray tube attached to a large C-shaped arm and you will be asked to lie on a table; something will be put under your head to support you. There are wires and cables and all sorts of technical terminology will be used by the staff and, although you may feel you are going to the electric chair or about to be operated on by Baron Frankenstein, you will, in the majority of cases, wonder what all the fuss was about when the procedure is finished.

A special tube called a *catheter* is put into the heart via an artery, either in the right elbow or, more usually nowadays, at the top of the right leg. If it is done from the elbow your arm will be laid out on to a special board and cleaned with antiseptic solution (which is cold). If it is done from the groin you will be shaved – you may do this yourself – and the antiseptic solution will be applied to that area. You will be draped with sterile green towels so the procedure is conducted exactly like an operation, with care taken not to introduce any infection. The doctor carrying out the test will be wearing a sterile gown and often a theatre hat and mask. He will be able to talk to you during the procedure.

Your ECG will be monitored during the test. A small amount of local anaesthetic is injected into the skin and the doctor should warn you when this is coming. This is usually no worse than having a dental anaesthetic injected into the gums. I have managed to train myself over the years to say 'you will feel a tiny injection in the skin', not 'you will feel a small prick in the groin' ...

A gentle doctor will usually trickle the anaesthetic medicine in slowly and ensure it has time to work. Once the area is numbed you should feel very little else. If the test is being done from the arm the doctor will make a small cut in the skin and spend a few minutes finding the artery which lies over the elbow joint. If it is done from the groin a small needle is put into the artery under the skin crease and a little tube or sheath passed into the artery. Once the catheter is introduced the cylindrical x-ray tube will sit over your chest. If it touches you or makes you feel uncomfortable, please tell the doctor or nurse. The doctor will then pass the catheter up, via the sheath, through your abdomen into your chest and round into your heart, while watching the x-ray screen. You will not feel any of this because, after all, you do not feel you blood going round, so you should not feel the tube going round.

The doctor will ask for various things to be done by the assistants and the x-ray tube will rotate around you – to your left hand side, back to the middle and then to the right. The doctor will turn the tip of the catheter while watching the x-ray monitor so he can see when the catheter goes into the coronary arteries. At this stage you might be asked to take a deep breath in and hold it and you may hear a whirring noise while the camera takes a picture. You will then be asked to breathe normally. Sometimes doctors forget to tell patients to breathe normally again so don't wait until you have turned blue – just breathe out when you feel like it!

Occasionally, while the dye is being injected down the artery patients may feel a slight burning sensation or tightness in the chest. This is nothing to worry about but do let the doctor know. Don't worry if you hear the technicians and nurses using unfamiliar terms such as 'left or right oblique'; it is all part of the routine. All we ask of you is that you lie as still as you can, breathe in and out when you are asked to and keep your arms still. People are often tempted to bring their left arm up over their chest but if you do that the doctor will end up with a nice x-ray picture of your hand!

At some stage the doctor will put one of the catheters directly into the pumping chamber of your heart. This may cause palpitations because when the tube touches the wall of the heart it makes it contract. An experienced doctor will warn you about this and will tell you not to worry about them. The main pumping chamber of the heart is then x-rayed by putting some dye into it. This enables us to see how well it is beating, whether there are any areas which don't move and whether any of the valves are leaking. When the dye goes in you will get a hot flush around your body as though you have just eaten a hot potato, and some people feel as if they have wet themselves because the dye spreads all over the body to all points. The doctor should warn you about the hot, flushing feeling and it won't last more than a few seconds.

In the early days of this test the dye used to make people sick but modern dyes are kinder and few patients feel unwell as it goes in. The procedure only lasts about 20-25 minutes and at the end you will either have someone pressing on your groin for a while to stop the bleeding or the doctor will put a few stitches in your arm. People often find that the pressure on the groin is the most uncomfortable part of the procedure but by that time they are usually so glad it's over that they don't mind.

Once the test is over, your arm or leg might start to throb a little as the local anaesthetic wears off but usually there is not much pain. You will be taken on a trolley, either to the ward or to a recovery area where a nurse will check your pulse rate, blood pressure and look for signs of bleeding. You will need to stay in bed for a few hours and then be allowed to go home. You should not drive yourself home nor go by public transport; it is best that you take a taxi or have a relation collect you.

My usual advice is that patients should go straight to bed and rest their arm or leg overnight to minimise any chance of late bleeding. Often a pressure dressing will have been applied to the groin – this can be soaked off in the bath the next day. If there are stitches in the arm these are usually self-dissolving.

You should be given an idea of what the results of the test are before you go home. Practices differ from consultant to consultant but someone fairly senior will normally look at the angiogram pictures and give you an idea of what they show. The consultant will later look at the pictures with his or her team and make a final decision.

A fairly recent innovation is the *mobile catheterisation laboratory* where the x-ray room is in the back of a van! The van may go to hospitals once a fortnight, allowing the local heart specialist to do a list of, say, a dozen patients. Not everyone in the profession is in favour of this because of concern about what would happen if the doctor needed to take the patient back to the laboratory later because of a complication, only to find that the lorry is 35 miles away!

Fortunately, complications of the angiogram are rare but occasionally the coronary arteries can go into spasm or be injured during the procedure. In a few cases, people with extreme narrowings may become unstable during the procedure and need to have the narrowing fixed immediately. Before the profession allows high-technology investigations to proliferate outside centres that handle large numbers of angiograms, we must think of the implications for patient safety. Although the angiogram is a safe procedure, complications will occur, however rarely.

The most common complications, however, do not arise from the heart but from the site where the tube was put into the artery. If you have had an angiogram done via your arm and your arm later becomes white or very painful you must contact the hospital immediately because it could mean that a blood clot has developed at the site where the artery was opened. I know of cases where people have not reported pain, thinking it normal, and have ended up having extensive surgery to their arms. Similarly, if your groin becomes swollen or bleeds, apply pressure and call the hospital. Some bruising of the groin may occur and sometimes this can look quite alarming. The skin of the groin and the leg might turn blue and purple but the bruising nearly always looks worse than it is, and will always disappear with time.

Remember that you can't have any procedure done, however minor, without the risk of some complication. Removal of a verruca or an in-growing toenail, or the injection of varicose veins, are fairly minor procedures but there is nevertheless a measurable complication rate, however small.

Others procedures performed in the laboratories include putting in pacemakers, biopsies of the heart muscle and special electrical stimulation tests performed on people with abnormal heart rhythms

WAITING AROUND

In an ideal world tests would be available straight away and in a few hospitals it is indeed possible to go straight from seeing the specialist to having an ultrasound scan and to be given the results immediately. This is obviously highly efficient and saves time. Most hospitals, however, do not have enough technical staff or equipment to be able to offer these 'one-stop' clinics and the likelihood is that you will be asked to come back for some of these tests. Waiting lists vary but it is not uncommon in big hospitals in busy cities to have to wait several weeks or months to have your investigations. This is not your doctor's fault so please don't phone up the secretary and hurl abuse when, having seen the consultant in January, you receive an appointment for your echo test in June or July.

My preferred practice is that if I don't think the tests are going to show anything horrific, I tell the patient that I will write to them with the results and only arrange to see them again if the test shows something unexpected. This is efficient for both the patient and for me as there is really no need to come to outpatients only to be told there is nothing wrong, when a letter will achieve the same result.

Heart specialists used to be regarded as successful if they had hundreds of outpatients queuing up to see them. Today, in the era of high technology heart specialists may spend less time in outpatients than they used to and more time doing tests or operating. If someone has been used to coming up to hospital once every three months to have their blood pressure taken, this responsibility can be delegated to the GP. Similarly, a patient with mild stable angina, controlled on tablets, does not really need to come up to tell the hospital doctor that he or she is feeling well. We rely on the GP to let us know if the patient's condition changes and then we take appropriate action.

Some patients find it hard to come to terms with being told they don't need repeated hospital check-ups, as they see it as a kind of safety net, a link with the hospital should they become ill. The reality is that patients are unlikely to be taken acutely ill on the day of their outpatient appointment and if illness occurs it will probably occur during the three months or so between appointments, when they will call their GP or an ambulance. We try to instil in patients a feeling that they have access to us at all times if necessary so they should not be frightened if we say they no longer need a routine appointment.

If a heart specialist decides that a patient should go on a waiting list for in-hospital investigations, the patient's position on the waiting list will be determined by his or her medical need.

Most patients have no idea of the machinations that go on in a cardiac centre which is coping with a large emergency referral base from outlying hospitals while trying to ensure that patients on the waiting list who are not emergencies also get treated. Bed closures around the country have made it increasingly difficult for hospital doctors to cope with their workload; having to push more and more patients through fewer and fewer hospital beds obviously causes immense difficulties. Although politicians like to point out that fewer patients wait eighteen months for treatment, the consequence of this is that patients in more urgent need end up waiting six to twelve months.

Although this will be no consolation to you if you are languishing on a waiting list, do remember that priorities change according to the clinical situation. For example, if an aeroplane suddenly has engine trouble 35,000 feet up, arrangements can be made for the plane to land at the nearest airport, even if this means keeping other planes waiting. A similar thing happens in medicine. If you are on a waiting list and your symptoms get worse, for goodness sake tell your GP or phone the consultant's secretary at the hospital. We do our best to respond and to expedite admission when things change, as they can do very rapidly in the case of heart problems.

CASUALTY

I have referred previously to the way patients may be admitted to hospital with heart pain or a heart attack, and your first encounter with a hospital may not be on a one-to-one basis in outpatients, but in the hubbub of a casualty department.

Those of you who are addicted to medical dramas on television might wonder if casualty staff spend all day gazing into each others' eyes while attending cardiac arrest calls. Have you noticed that at Holby General Hospital patients are not parked on trolleys for hours? This may be politically correct but, unfortunately, the reality is very different.

Many casualty departments have their cubicles full of patients who have waited hours for beds to become available; remaining patients are parked on trolleys which are scattered at various angles like cars in a motorway pile-up. In these conditions it is sometimes difficult to maintain basic human dignities and privacy. It is difficult to know how to advise people about the best way to behave in casualty but there is no point complaining to the overworked doctors and nursing staff. It is not their fault that neighbouring casualty departments have closed and their workload increased; nor is it their fault that there is a shortage of beds, in spite of what politicians may say.

Sometimes if a patient with heart pain has been waiting in casualty all night he or she may have a visit from the heart specialist in casualty on the morning ward round. People are often impressed by the fact that they are visited by a specialist before they even have a bed found for them!

I came across an article in a popular American magazine. The amusing advice it contained may be applicable to a small proportion of the American public but would be difficult to implement in the war zones that are most

British casualty departments. The advice included:

Make sure your physician supports the aggressive use of clot-buster drugs.

I can't imagine terrified patients lying there clutching their chests, sweating profusely yet interrogating their doctor about whether he or she is familiar with the use of the clot-buster drugs!

Choose the best hospital.

The article pointed out that in one American state there were big differences in the time taken to administer the clot-buster drugs and patients were advised to ensure that they are taken to the hospital with the best track record.

In the UK, where stories abound of heart attack victims being refused admission (in one case by up to nine hospitals) because of lack of beds, it is hard not to smile at a Michelin-type guide for patients advising them calmly – in the middle of their heart attack – to instruct the ambulance driver 'Take me to St Elsewhere's.'

Carry your electrocardiogram with you. Photocopy it down to fit in your wallet.

The theory behind this is sound, in as much as if the doctor in casualty can see what your ECG looked like before you had your pain and then compare it with the one taken during pain it may be easier to make a diagnosis. However, the practicalities involved in asking patients to carry copies of their ECGs around with them in their wallets make the mind boggle. I can just imagine the patient, in the middle of a heart attack, asking the ambulance man to wait while they find their wallet!

Be assertive in the emergency room.

If there is one place where people feel at their most vulnerable and least assertive it is in the middle of a casualty department. Can you see a heart attack victim in a busy casualty department saying, 'Now look here my good man – I believe I'm having a heart attack. Please attend to me immediately and administer a clot-buster drug without delay or I shall speak to your superior!'

Finally:

You can call in a cardiologist for a second opinion.

Whereas it may be a bit much to expect the casualty department to summon up a cardiologist like a genie from a bottle, if you have a heart problem and have not seen a heart specialist you should do your utmost to see one at some stage, sooner rather than later.

In the next chapter I will go through the treatments that are available once the results of all the investigations have been assessed and I will discuss the way you can participate in making informed choices about what treatments are best for you.

10

IT'S TIME TO FIX THE PLUMBING
TREATMENTS OF HEART DISEASE

DOCTOR: Well, I've now got the results of your tests, Mrs Jones, so we shall discuss the treatment.

MRS JONES: Yes, doctor.

DOCTOR: We're just going to chop your head off, dice your body up into small pieces, stick it into plastic bags and shove you out of the window.

MRS JONES: Anything you say, doctor.

This extract from a student Christmas ward show may be an exaggeration, but it makes the point that the public have blind faith in their medical advisers and rarely question the treatment which is offered to them. Things have changed, however, and doctors have found their pedestals knocked askew as patients realise that doctors are mere mortals and as the media highlight with 'shock horror' headlines every mistake a doctor makes.

In cardiology we do have a tendency to be technology-driven and, as a new piece of gee-whizz equipment becomes available, the indications to use that toy proliferate rapidly. We need to think hard about the risks and benefits of any treatment and to restrain ourselves from using the latest gizmo just because we want to be the first to do so.

The latest buzz phrase among medical economists is

'evidence-based medicine'. This term seeks to invoke best medical practice whereby doctors abandon medical or technological treatments which have been shown to be ineffective and only use therapies which are of proven efficacy. At one extreme anyone would think we were still applying leeches or doling out medicines brewed on some blasted heath by the three witches in Shakespeare's *Macbeth*! At the other extreme is the notion that every treatment has been subjected to rigorous scientific examination in laboratory-controlled conditions in highly selected populations.

Protagonists of evidence-based medicine believe that doctors will tap into a computer and find out what evidence is available before deciding on an appropriate treatment. The Catch 22 in the practice of evidence-based medicine is that a certain treatment cannot be used unless it has been proved effective – but how can one prove it effective without using it first? Not every question in medicine has been answered scientifically by clinical trials with statistical analyses.

Opponents of evidence-based medicine point out that if a doctor has been working for several years in general practice or in a speciality, he or she will have a vast wealth of experience and will have a 'feel' which cannot be taught, and a clinical experience which cannot be printed out by a computer.

As usual, truth probably lies half way between the two extremes. GPs and specialists must keep themselves up to date with the latest advances and must be familiar with the results of trials which show whether a treatment is effective or has been superseded by a more modern approach.

One of the great fears of moving towards a computerised treatment plan is that it will permit purchasing authorities to refuse to pay for treatments which are regarded by these authorities as ineffective. The furore over a health authority's refusal to treat the little girl known as 'Child B' highlights this. Who is to say, for example, that if the treatment she eventually received for her leukaemia buys her another five years of life, an absolute cure won't be found within that five-year period?

The arguments apply especially to heart disease which is so common and where analysis of cost places extreme pressure on specialists to choose one form of treatment over another. It may be cheap for a purchasing authority to have Mrs Jones diced into pieces but it would hardly be in her best interests!

It is important that patients understand not only what is wrong with them but what the treatment advised entails, what alternatives there are, and why one particular treatment is recommended. Good communication is of paramount importance.

A critic wrote recently: 'The next set of hospital wards to re-open ought to be devoted to image transplants for the medical establishment, a body which is suffering from rigor mortis of the communication joints ... the medical establishment regards itself as having sole access to that which is good for us and will be sure to let us know when and if some suitable tablet can be brought down from the mountain.' (*Daily Telegraph*, February 1996)

What the critic overlooked is that the majority of patients want their doctor to tell them what is good for them because they don't know themselves. For example, I know nothing abut the intricate workings of my car engine. If it goes wrong I want it fixed by someone I can trust and I don't necessarily want to be presented with the results of scientific research projects in order to decide whether my car needs a new water pump, or whether the brake linings need to be renewed.

This notwithstanding, there is a difference between a replaceable motor car and an irreplaceable body. Our capacity to interfere with disease processes by high-powered drugs and to develop seemingly endless high-technology gadgets with which to invade the body have led people to question what on earth doctors are up to. Trust in doctors is one thing, blind unquestioning faith is another.

With heart problems, things are often not clear cut and for any condition even experienced and competent cardiologists have different opinions over the treatment to be prescribed. Such differences don't necessarily mean that one cardiologist is wrong and the other right: different advice can often be equally well justified. It is a question of whether or not the doctor is able to communicate what the choices are and why one particular strategy is recommended over another.

The patient must have an input as well, if they want one. Some people will have good reasons for wanting to avoid, say, major heart surgery, while other patients will be more keen on an interventionist approach. If patient and doctor understand each other the treatment process can proceed calmly.

When a doctor sets out to treat angina, for example, the objective is to control the patient's symptoms. However, treatment of angina is only one part of the strategy of treating furred-up arteries. Unfortunately, there is no cure for coronary artery disease at the moment – it is not like having a gall bladder full of stones or appendicitis where, with a few slick slices, the surgeon can remove the offending bit and the problem won't recur.

The symptoms of angina can be helped by attending to lifestyle matters such as losing weight if possible and giving up smoking as well as having blood pressure or a high cholesterol level treated where appropriate. I am always amazed at the number of patients who claim to eat absolutely nothing yet fail to lose weight, defying all known science. I can recall a conversation with a rotund

Greek man from North London who swore to me that he consumed no food at all and yet remained around 20 stone.

ME: I just don't see how that's possible.

PATIENT: It's the truth, doctor.

At this point his wife, who had been bristling in the corner, felt compelled to speak.

WIFE: Tell the truth! Last night there were three loaves of bread in the larder and this morning there is only one. Where are the other two?

PATIENT: Well – I woke up in the middle of the night and I was peckish so I came down for a snack.

ME AND WIFE: (simultaneously) A snack? Two loaves of bread?!

PATIENT: Well, OK. I don't eat anything apart from the occasional loaf of bread!

I have had similar discussions with a learned rabbi and his wife about exactly how many bagels and pickled cucumbers he was allowed to consume in one day. I couldn't be too hard on him; after all, these are some of my life's great pleasures too.

Specific treatment for the syndromes produced by furred-up arteries consists of suppressing the symptoms and deciding whether anything can be done to prevent premature death. Treatment is thus both symptomatic and prognostic. Strategies for treating symptoms are fairly easy to comprehend but those aimed at prolonging life are more difficult and controversial. Let me deal with the easy bit first.

DRUG TREATMENTS FOR ANGINA

As I explained earlier, angina, or cramp from the heart muscle, occurs when demand for oxygen exceeds supply. In order to redress the balance we can either reduce the amount of oxygen the heart needs or we can increase its supply. As a general rule medical treatment with tablets reduces the demand for oxygen and surgical treatment will increase supply. Medical treatment can be further subdivided into treatment of the acute attack and prevention of future attacks.

GTN

Many people who suffer from angina know that the treatment of an acute attack of angina involves putting a tablet or a spray under the tongue. This medication is known as *glyceryl trinitrate*, often shortened to *GTN*. It reduces the amount of oxygen the heart needs, thus restoring the balance.

GTN usually works quickly, although with the following provisos. First, GTN tablets lose their effectiveness after a few months, so always keep a fresh supply. Secondly, if the tablet doesn't dissolve it can't do much good, so if your mouth is dry moisten it – in these circumstances the spray may be preferable. Thirdly, one of the side-effects is a pounding headache as the arteries around the body dilate. Also, remember that if you know that a certain activity, such as climbing uphill or walking in a stiff breeze brings on the pain you can use the tablet before you set out to try to prevent the pain starting.

GTN tablets are not addictive and they are short-acting. You shouldn't worry if you need to use three or four a day. However, if this is the only treatment you are on and you are shovelling GTN tablets into your mouth like Smarties, you should certainly be on some other tablets to try to prevent the attacks. Such tablets are called *anti-anginal medications*. I cannot go into the details of every proprietary medicine that is available for angina but I will mention the various groups of drugs.

Beta-blockers

Perhaps the commonest to be used are the beta-blocker drugs. These slow the heart rate down, reduce blood pressure and reduce the work the heart has to do with each beat. The combined effect is to lessen the amount of oxygen the heart needs. Beta-blockers come in all shapes and sizes. Some are taken once a day and others may be taken three or four times a day. Beta-blockers are commonly prescribed after an uncomplicated heart attack but can't be given to people if they have a very damaged heart muscle which would be weakened further, or if they have severe bronchitis or asthma because they can narrow the airways. If someone has narrowed arteries in the legs and pain in the back of their calves when they walk, beta-blockers can make this worse.

Calcium blockers

Another set of drugs which are often used are called *calcium blockers* and many of these need only to be taken once a day. Calcium blockers open up the arteries around the body and may cause a sensation of feeling flushed. Some of them slow the heart rate more than others, but they all reduce the amount of work the heart has to do. One side-effect specific to these drugs is that they can cause ankle swelling.

Nitrates

The third major group of drugs are long-acting versions of

the tablet which you can put under your tongue, collectively known as *nitrates*. There are a whole variety of these available but they all have the same side-effect of causing a headache in some people.

These drugs don't have to be used alone and some people with angina are on beta-blockers and calcium blockers or various other combinations. When one is on all three drugs this is known as triple therapy. These days any patients with angina would also be on a small daily dose of aspirin because of its beneficial effects in stopping blood clotting.

You should know that any drug can cause any side-effects in patients and that sometimes individual reactions to these drugs are unpredictable. It is unlikely that any of them will make you sprout antlers or turn your hair green but they can cause skin rashes and nausea in some people. If you are experiencing side-effects please let your doctor know because there will usually be an alternative treatment which won't have the same effects.

Whether or not you end up on triple therapy and sucking GTN tablets without seeing a heart specialist will depend largely on the attitude of your GP to referring you to a specialist. A very conservative specialist may only offer the series of tests leading up to the angiogram if your symptoms are persistent despite taking tablets, whereas another specialist with a different attitude towards the management of furred-up arteries will arrange for you to have the tests even if your symptoms are mild.

SURGERY FOR ANGINA

Most heart specialists faced with a patient who is still having symptoms in spite of tablets, will consider whether there is any alternative to medication. There is no reason why anybody should put up with terrible angina or take twenty pills a day to control it without at least having the benefit of a full assessment to see whether some sort of surgical approach might help. There are patients who have gone through the whole gamut of tests but are not suitable for anything other than tablets, either because the arteries are too bad or because they have other illnesses which would make a surgical approach too dangerous. The conscientious GP or specialist will weigh up these external factors before suggesting any intervention.

If you have bad angina that is not being controlled properly by tablets you should ask for something to be done if it is not being offered to you. Books with such titles as *Coping with Angina* may make people believe that there is no way of getting rid of it but that is not the case.

Since the early 1980s the technology whereby cardiologists can deal with furred-up arteries with the patient awake has snowballed in what amounts to a cardiological Big Bang. Cardiologists have changed from being solely doctors who diagnose conditions to those who undertake procedures to deal with narrowings and these doctors are broadly termed *interventional cardiologists.*

It is currently very sexy to be an interventional cardiologist. Most young doctors in training want to become familiar with the paraphernalia and feel left out if they only do outpatient clinics, echo scans and maybe a few angiograms. If you were to watch heart specialists attending some of the major international conferences such as the American Heart Association or the European Society of Cardiology, you would see cardiologists running towards a session on interventional cardiology like wildebeests stampeding across the plains of Kenya. In order to get a place in the seminar room you may have to be there two hours early. Meanwhile in an adjacent hall some poor research worker is presenting his latest work on a rat with high blood pressure to an audience of two or three!

Whereas tablets reduce the heart's demand for oxygen, the aim of surgery is to increase supply, either by opening up the narrowed segment of artery with a balloon or by having a by-pass operation.

Balloons

Balloon-related technology is known by the collective term of *angioplasty*, which means altering the shape of an artery. I will try to unravel some of the mysteries surrounding angioplasty. I must clarify some misconceptions about the word 'balloon'. First, this is not a balloon in the conventional, party sense: it is a small oval shaped balloon-like structure bonded to the tip of a fine tube or catheter. The balloon is transparent and made of a tough material called polyethylene.

When the catheter is taken out of its packet this balloon is wrapped closely around the shaft of the catheter. The reason it is tightly wrapped is because the balloon has to cross the narrowing in the artery, and the slimmer the balloon the easier it is to cross a very tight restriction in the coronary artery. A special inflation device full of fluid is attached to the other end of the catheter and when high pressure is applied to this fluid the small balloon expands. When expanded it is about 2 cm long and oval in shape. The balloons come in various widths because coronary arteries are not all the same size. These polyethylene balloons are designed to withstand about twelve times atmospheric pressure and they squash the obstructive goo against the artery walls.

Imagine a piece of dough shaped like a small hillock to represent the obstruction in the artery (see diagram on page 29). If with both hands you exert as much pressure as you can on top of the dough you will compress it and change its shape completely so it no longer sticks up. This is what the balloon does inside your artery. Obviously I have over-simplified this procedure but the principle of re-modelling the narrowing and compressing the obstruction up against the wall of the artery is one which should be quite easy to understand.

The technique used to introduce the balloon into the artery is much the same as that for the angiogram, with nearly all cardiologists inserting it through the groin. Sometimes patients are given medicine about an hour before the procedure to relax them. This is called a *pre-med*.

The next trick is to put all the hardware into the relevant artery. If you look back at the diagrams you may find it difficult to understand how we can navigate down this complex network of arteries and control where we are going. The first step is to take a very fine guide wire, usually about 14,000th inch in diameter, and with one's fingertips make a small bend on the tip. With the help of the x-ray tube and small injections of dye we can turn and twist the wire so that it goes down the correct artery. This requires very fine finger movements as the wire must be passed down gently to avoid damaging the inside of the artery.

While the wire is being manipulated into the coronary tree you should not experience discomfort and may wonder whether anything is happening at all. Some patients find it interesting to watch what is happening on the screen while others wish they weren't there at all and keep their eyes screwed tightly shut. I find it often helps if the doctor or an assistant explains to the patient what is happening.

Once the wire is positioned across the obstruction, the balloon catheter is fed over the wire and placed across the narrowing. The balloon is then gently inflated with fluid through the inflation device. The size of balloon used will depend on the operator's judgement on the width of the artery. Most arteries are between 2.5 and 3.5 mm wide, which is really quite small, and the only way we can see what we are doing is by having the x-ray tube magnify the heart to give us a decent-sized picture.

When the balloon is inflated you might experience some chest discomfort because the balloon blocks off the artery for a minute or so and makes the muscle short of blood. It is absolutely normal to experience some chest discomfort, but someone should warn you that it is coming. It should ease when the balloon is deflated and the discomfort is usually tolerable. The specialist will use injections of dye to check that the narrowing has gone away.

Sometimes only two or three inflations of the balloon are necessary but occasionally material in the artery is quite tough and requires more work. The cardiologist has to judge how hard he or she strives to achieve a picture that looks perfect, or when discretion is the better part of valour. The aim is a patient who will be free of angina, hopefully in the long term, and not necessarily a perfect-looking artery.

Achieving a good result takes experience and careful judgement on the specialist's part. However, not all doctors who carry out angioplasty have the chance to do enough operations to maintain their skills – you wouldn't expect Michael Schumacher to do one Grand Prix race a year and maintain his edge as a world champion driver, or Eric Cantona to play six football matches a year and keep his fitness and skills.

Balloon technology has evolved dramatically over the last 15 years and I shudder to think of what we used when we first started in 1980. Today these catheters are very high-tech pieces of equipment indeed. They have become thinner and thinner which enables them to get through difficult obstructions but they must be robust enough not to buckle when the doctor advances them, but to stay straight and track down the wire.

If you are lying there listening to the doctors you may be amused – or alarmed – at requests for 'a 3.5 Falcon' or a 'Cat'. These balloons have wonderful names to reflect the sleekness of the products (the manufacturers no doubt have highly paid marketing people who sit for days dreaming them up). We also have Panthers, Cobras and Cheetahs, Sambas, Prontos and Rallies, Expresses and Speedies. We have an Atlantis and a Europass – which sounds like an identity card dreamt up by Brussels. We even have a Predator, which is all right as long as it doesn't turn into a Terminator! Given that the balloons are getting thinner and thinner I am disappointed that my own suggestions of an Anorexic, a Skeleton or a Ghost have not been taken up. The specialist will use the balloon technology with which he or she is most familiar and which will provide the best result. In practice most balloons will deal with the majority of narrowings quite effectively.

As we are dealing with delicate arteries it is inevitable that complications will sometimes arise. Occasionally the artery might block off completely during the procedure, either because of a tear caused during passage of the balloon or its inflation or because a blood clot forms. However, complications are rare and run in the region of 1–2 per cent of cases. Recent developments have made it much easier to cope with these problems but occasionally, although rarely, the heart muscle might be damaged during the procedure.

Angioplasty is nearly always carried out with what is known as *surgical cover* which means that there is a heart surgeon nearby in case the artery rebels at having wires and balloons put down it and won't open up. If the specialist thinks that the problem cannot be solved the patient may have to have a by-pass operation there and then but this is unusual. With modern technology the need for such emergency by-pass surgery is diminishing. The overwhelming majority of patients have an uncomplicated angioplasty and are much better symptomatically after the procedure.

Before you have an angioplasty the doctor should discuss with you what is going to happen, what you should feel, and mention the surgical cover that is provided. Certain heart specialists around the world now believe you can do angioplasty without surgical cover but at the time of writing this is still the minority view. Even doing what is considered to be a low-risk narrowing, sod's law will dictate that if you don't have surgical cover available you will wish you had.

Patients often ask me whether bits of material can break off from the wall of the artery and block off the artery further down. This does happen but again it is extremely rare. Other patients ask whether the balloon is left inside the artery. It is not! Once the balloon has done its job it is removed.

Afterwards, different doctors will handle their patients in varying ways. Some will leave the little tubes in the groin overnight while the blood is thinned with a medicine called heparin dripping in through a vein. The reason for this is that if the artery misbehaves at three o'clock in the morning and we have to take the patient back to the x-ray room the tubes are already in place and we can get back into the artery very quickly. Other specialists like to get the tubes out of the groin as quickly as possible. Either way, if all goes well you should be in hospital for no more than a couple of nights and the great thing about angioplasty is that there is no real convalescence period and once your leg is no longer sore you can go back to work.

Angioplasty has had a bad press recently and the Chinese whispers that invariably accompany this procedure indicate that everybody has to have another angioplasty six months later. This isn't the case. There is no doubt that the Achilles heel of angioplasty is a recurrence of the narrowing. The jargon for this is *restenosis*. The exact instance of restenosis depends on how one defines it. Most of the research trials have carried out repeat angiograms six months down the line and shown that the artery may have renarrowed a little bit. There may be a 40–50 per cent narrowing at the site of the angioplasty whereas there may have been a 90–95 per cent narrowing before one started.

This may not actually matter. If the degree of renarrowing is not enough to cause symptoms or to put the patient at risk, and if the narrowing stays at 50 per cent and does not get any worse then we may be worrying unnecessarily. What is important is the number of patients who come back with recurrent symptoms and have to be redone. Between 25–30 per cent have to have a second go – which means that 70–75 per cent of patients don't!

There is much research being carried out to try to solve the problem of renarrowing and it will probably require some sort of drug therapy to stop the inner lining of the artery from furring up. There are some promising things on the horizon and most of us are quite confident that the problem will be solved eventually. If the procedure does have to be done again, however, the majority of patients will get a good result from the second angioplasty and avoid a by-pass operation. The beauty of angioplasty is that it can be repeated quite easily and, although no one wants to have needles stuck in their groin any more often than is necessary, this may still be preferable to having a by-pass operation which requires a longer hospital stay and period of recuperation.

Who should have an angioplasty as opposed to a by-pass operation? There is a polarisation of views on this. These range from the evangelical cardiologist who thinks 'the only indication for a by-pass operation is a failed angioplasty', to the more sanguine approach that certain patients might be expected to do very well with angio-plasty and some will do better with a by-pass operation. As a rule if only one of the three major arteries is narrowed we do our best to avoid a by-pass operation. If all three arter-ies are narrowed surgery probably wins, because if there are too many narrowings to open up with a balloon the risk of some of them recurring is too high. Patients with two narrowed arteries may do very well with ballooning or surgery, but given the almost infinite combinations of blockages and narrowings, decisions have to be made on an individual basis every time.

Other widening techniques

Over the last few years newer techniques have evolved to attack coronary narrowings. These include balloons with blades on them which cut out the deposits on the wall, high-speed and low-speed drills, a device like a vacuum cleaner which hoovers up the goo, a whole host of laser technology to fry away the deposits, and small pieces of metal called *stents* which are used to hold the artery open after ballooning.

I cannot describe here how all these devices work and their advantages and disadvantages, except to say that however exciting it may be to try out these new devices they do not always work well.

There is something about the word laser which captures the public imagination. Because laser technology has been so successful in cutting away some cancers and in sealing back the retina when it becomes detached in the eye, patients often wonder why laser technology has not taken the heart by storm. Unfortunately it has not proved to be the universal cure for furred-up arteries.

A few years ago the cardiac conferences were full of talks on lasers but the jury is still out. The early attempts with lasers produced many complications and injury to the arterial wall, and because the laser beam has been difficult to control holes in the artery occurred accidentally – which could be disastrous. Laser technology has been more successful in dealing with blocked arteries in the legs than the heart. Such treatment may come to fruition eventually but at the moment it is of limited use so we shall just have to wait and see. The fact that your doctor doesn't offer you a *zap* and a *pow* for your narrowed arteries does not mean that he or she is out of date!

The one piece of new technology which is very promising and is used widely is the metallic *stent*. Basically, this a high-tech biro spring! It consists of a metal lattice or mesh which is mounted on the balloon catheter. As the balloon expands the stent is pushed right up against the wall where it acts as a piece of scaffolding, holding the artery open. Stents have made angioplasty easier because if the artery tears during the balloon procedure (a tear is known as a *dissection* and can obstruct the artery) it is nearly always possible now to put in a stent which pushes back the tear and restores the artery to normal. This has been described as wallpapering the artery. Metallic stents have reduced the need for emergency by-pass surgery.

Unlike the balloon, the stent is left inside the artery permanently and after a few weeks or months a lining of cells covers it, incorporating it into the wall of the artery. As well as being used to 'bail out' when balloon angioplasty becomes complicated, there is now a move to put stents in straight away in certain arteries. Research has shown that the incidence of renarrowing (restenosis) is less with stents than with ordinary ballooning and at six months follow-up this seems to be the case. We don't yet know whether we can solve renarrowing altogether by shoving a piece of metal into the artery or whether this just delays the renarrowing by a year or so. Time will tell.

On the horizon are a whole host of new developments including stents coated with drugs to try to stop the wall of the artery furring up again. We won't know if these work for some years to come. When stents were first used everybody put their patients on to blood-thinning drugs for a few months. Now there is a slight shift away from using warfarin towards other drugs which stop cells (called platelets) in the blood from sticking together and causing blood clots. These platelet cells are what stop us bleeding when we cut ourselves.

The whole field is changing rapidly, and no doubt by the year 2010 we will look back on what we are doing today as fairly primitive but it is unlikely that in my working lifetime heart disease will be treatable by the methods used by Dr McCoy in *Star Trek*.

By-pass surgery

Given that coronary heart disease is progressive it is probably sensible to regard angioplasty and the related technologies as a way of postponing by-pass surgery, hopefully indefinitely. Most of us who have been doing angioplasty for over ten years will have patients going back to the early 1980s who have had one procedure and no further trouble. Unfortunately, new narrowings crop up in arteries which were previously normal. If someone who has had an angioplasty comes back with a recurrent problem a year or more after the procedure it is more likely they have a new narrowing elsewhere than a recurrence of the old problem.

Heart surgeons often take a rather dim view of angioplasty but they shouldn't because there are still plenty of patients for them to chop up. This is particularly so in the UK where patients are often referred late on with advanced heart disease, and may be beyond the scope of ballooning.

Coronary artery by-pass surgery is now one of the most common operations performed. It is a major heart operation and as such is not to be recommended lightly. However, for people who have severely diseased arteries and whose heart pump is working normally the risk of not surviving the operation is about 1 per cent; 99 patients out of 100 will survive. In cases where the pump of the heart is damaged the risks are higher. Also, if the carotid arteries, which take blood to the brain, are narrowed the risks of the operation increase and the doctor has to weigh up the risks and benefits of surgery versus those of leaving well alone.

Most people do extremely well with a by-pass. This is a relatively simple plumbing procedure using a new pipe to by-pass a blocked one. The operation consists of taking a piece of vein (called a *saphenous vein*) from the leg, starting at or around the ankle and, depending how much vein is needed, going up to just below the knee or into the thigh. The vein is carefully taken out and inspected to make sure it is of good quality. The vein in then turned round. The reason for this is that the veins in the legs have valves in them which stop the blood falling back towards the feet. Just like the valves in the heart they permit the blood to flow only one way. The surgeon therefore has to ensure that the blood can flow in the right direction!

Patients often ask how it is possible to have a vein taken from the leg without this preventing the blood getting back from the leg to the heart. The answer is that the veins used are superficial ones which lie close to the skin. There is an enormous network of superficial and deep veins that one can't see and so that even if a vein is taken away the blood will find its way back to the deep veins and back to the heart, in the same way as an experienced cab driver who finds the main roads blocked will get around using the 'back doubles'.

One end of the vein is stitched to the aorta, and the other

end is stitched to the coronary artery beyond the blockage. For the artery down the front of the heart, or left anterior descending, good long-term results are obtained by using an artery which sits in the chest called the *left internal mammary artery*, often shortened to *lima*. This artery branches off the main artery that goes towards the arm and its only function is to supply blood to the chest wall and to the breast. For this reason it is often known as the 'boob tube'! The surgeon will carefully tease out the artery, swing it down and stitch it on to the coronary artery.

The diagram opposite shows what vein by-passes and an internal mammary by-pass look like; the arrows show the direction the blood is flowing through the by-passes.

The internal mammary artery tends to stay open longer than vein by-passes. The problem with veins is that, although they may give very good symptomatic relief for anything from eight to fifteen years, they were not actually designed to carry blood at the speed at which arteries do, and for some reason the veins gradually fur up over a period of years. People who continue smoking, have high cholesterol or bad diabetes are likely to find the vein by-passes do not last as long as they do in people without these risk factors. Some promising new research has suggested new ways of keeping vein by-passes open longer.

Any patient undergoing a surgical procedure will need to sign a consent form. This contains a description of the operation and states that the patient understands what the procedure entails and that he or she agrees to a local or general anaesthetic. In the past a patient who needed a by-pass would have a visit from an eminent consultant who would speak to him as if he were senile: 'You need an operation, old boy,' the Grand Old Man would say, patting the patient's knee, 'it'll make you better.' End of explanation. However, as what you are asked to sign is called *informed consent*, don't sign it unless you have read the form care-

Diagram to show how the left internal mammary artery, and veins from the legs, are used in a coronary by-pass operation to 'by-pass' the obstructions

The aorta

Vein by-pass graft on to the right coronary artery

Left internal mammary artery (lima) by-pass to left anterior descending

Vein by-passes to circumflex branches

221

fully and understand what you are going through.

Heart by-passes are done under deep anaesthesia. While the surgeon operates, a machine takes over the function of the heart, pumping the blood round the body and keeping the brain and the kidneys supplied with oxygen. Patients come out of the operating theatre into the *intensive care unit (ICU)*, where they are kept on a breathing machine for a while but encouraged to wake up and breathe on their own as quickly as possible. Most people stay in hospital after a by-pass operation for 7–10 days.

The most common complications are usually chest infections – especially in smokers – or small areas of collapsed lung which require time and physiotherapy to expand again. Rhythm disturbances, particularly in the heart's filling chambers (atrial fibrillation), can occur a day or two after heart surgery but they nearly always settle down with the appropriate drugs and they are rarely a long-term problem.

Sometimes patients become a little confused after heart surgery, especially if they have spent a while in intensive care, where it is often difficult to tell the difference between night and day and nurses buzz around the patient like wasps around a jam jar. I remember one patient who refused to let the physiotherapist see him because he had read her name badge as 'PHYSIO THE RAPIST'.

The physio is probably the most important person involved in helping people recover from heart surgery, using exercises to expand the lungs and helping the patient become mobile. The majority of patients will go home after seven days with a cold nose, a glossy coat and a wagging tail. Some people will need a longer hospital stay because of infection, rhythm problems or, worst of all, a stroke after the operation.

It is awful for everybody if a patient has a stroke after heart surgery. This is usually caused by sludge from the aorta which breaks off during the operation and gets stuck in the brain. We take all the precautions we can. In older patients, we ensure that the arteries that supply the brain are clear by scanning them with ultrasound. Most people will recover after a stroke but a very unfortunate minority will be left with some sort of disability. Let me stress that strokes are unusual and let me remind you that any operation, be it ever so minor, carries the risk of some complication.

People are generally off work for four to six weeks after the operation and it is surprising how quickly the leg and chest wounds heal up and the need for painkillers diminishes. The odd healing pain may persist in the chest for a few months but these aches are usually not too troublesome. We expect people to get back to work and complete normality in the vast majority of cases.

Wherever possible, the doctor should try to involve the patient in the decision-making process, although not like this:

CONSULTANT: Mr Harris, your coronary angiogram shows severe proximal stenoses in two of your major coronary vessels and a moderate lesion in the third.

MR HARRIS: Really, doctor?

CONSULTANT: Yes, there is marked arteriosclerosis in the entire arterial tree.

MR HARRIS: Oh dear, doctor.

CONSULTANT: We have two possible treatment strategies for you. We can either undertake a double vessel balloon angioplasty, which we might do as a staged procedure ...

223

MR HARRIS: Yes, doctor.

CONSULTANT: Or we might do both lesions at the same sitting depending on how we get on and leave the least severe stenosis.

MR HARRIS: If you think that's a good idea doctor ...

CONSULTANT: Or alternatively, we could recommend full revascularisation with a triple coronary by-pass operation.

MR HARRIS: I see, doctor.

CONSULTANT: Good. Have a think about it and I'll see you in outpatients.

You may think that no doctor could possibly talk to a patient like this but sometimes they do. Nurses often have to go around mopping up after consultants, translating what they have said into English!

The preferences of a patient must be considered. Some people will do anything to avoid having their chest split open whereas others would rather have a big operation and get the whole thing out of the way at once.

A by-pass is not a cure. Although research has shown that there is less requirement for second operations in the early stages after by-pass surgery compared to angioplasty, people do come back some years down the line with recurrent problems. The younger you are when you have a by-pass operation, the more likely you are to require something else doing twelve or fifteen years later. Although attention to risk factors is important there is little we can do at present to stop the veins wearing out. Many people require a second or even a third by-pass operation. If the veins from the legs have all been used up on the first operation then arm veins may be used instead. Balloon related technology can be applied to furred-up veins quite successfully and is a useful way of buying time and avoiding a further operation.

If a patient comes back with recurrent angina and is shown on an angiogram to have a tight narrowing in the vein by-pass it can be ballooned open and a stent implanted. Quite often this will solve the problem. Recurrent problems are more common in old by-passes which become clogged up with sludge. Sometimes if a blood clot develops in the vein by-pass it can be cleared with a clot-buster drug.

Heart surgeons like to operate on virgin chests and are less keen to take on a patient for a second operation. Even allowing for technological improvements, the risks of a second by-pass are greater than the first operation. This is because the surgeon has to cut through all the scar tissue and the operation may take longer.

After a by-pass operation the patient will be seen in outpatients by the surgeon who will want to check his needle-work and by the cardiologist who will want to make sure that risk factors are being modified and that there are no residual 'i's to be dotted and 't's to be crossed. Patients often come back to outpatients not feeling 100 per cent, but to be walking two or three miles a day, a few weeks after a major heart operation is quite an achievement and I advise patients that the healing process may take months. I always tell patients they will have good days and bad days once they get home but that the good days will become more frequent and the bad days rarer.

Alternative techniques

It is worth mentioning some of the alternative techniques for treating angina in patients who are unsuitable for either balloon treatment or an ordinary by-pass operation.

Some years ago there was a vogue for implanting a

device next to the spinal cord which the patient could activate when they had an anginal attack and which would stimulate a nerve to try to alleviate the pain. This device is called a *dorsal column stimulator*, but it hasn't really caught on and is very expensive.

Currently, experimental work is taking place which uses a laser (yes, that device again) to punch tiny holes in the heart muscle and create little lakes of blood in the middle of the muscle fibres. We jokingly call this the 'crocodile operation' because the hearts of reptiles get their blood supply from lagoons like this inside the heart muscle. This procedure tries to create the same effect in human beings. Initial reports have been encouraging but then early reports of new techniques usually are. The procedure needs to be tested vigorously before we raise people's hopes and expectations too far.

THE PROBLEM OF MISSING SYMPTOMS

I have so far talked about treating symptoms but I should also talk about treatment to increase life expectancy. As I have said earlier the workload of most heart specialists is so great that they can only treat people who have bad symptoms. This should not stop us striving to deal with life-threatening conditions which don't cause too many symptoms. After all, if a woman is unfortunate enough to have breast cancer diagnosed at a routine examination because someone feels a lump we don't just leave it, do we? Equally, treating high blood pressure is a benefit yet most people with this condition don't have symptoms. So why should we treat the coronary arteries any differently?

Since the mid-1970s a lot of work has been done to try to assess which people are at risk from major heart attacks. Nearly all cardiologists would agree that if a patient has narrowing of the left main artery (see diagram on page 29) then surgery is indicated, even if symptoms are mild, because the chances of survival without surgery are low. Similarly, if all three major arteries have severe narrowings and especially if the pumping ability of the heart is slightly impaired, current evidence suggests that patients benefit from by-pass surgery. Beyond these groups, however, cardiologists will argue several sets of hind legs off a herd of donkeys about who should and should not have treatment on life-expectancy grounds instead of symptoms.

At one stage in the late 1970s life seemed fairly straightforward because research showed that the greater the number of narrowed arteries the worse the survival. This was later extended to show that by-pass surgery conferred no benefit on life expectancy in patients with one narrowed artery, some benefit in patients with two narrowed arteries and a great deal of benefit in patients with three narrowed arteries. It therefore seemed quite easy to practise cardiology by counting the number of narrow tubes on the angiogram and recommending tablets or by-pass surgery accordingly.

Since then we have been forced to put our brains back into gear as it has become apparent that not all patients with one narrowed artery do well without surgery and some will come to grief, and that not every patient with three narrowed arteries will do badly without an operation. What was needed was some way of assessing the impact of the narrowing on the heart muscle. The simplest technique was the treadmill test.

Much effort has gone into attempting to use the treadmill test to predict the future and, as usual, the published evidence is conflicting. Current wisdom is that if a patient with three narrowed arteries can do 15 minutes on the treadmill and achieve a barnstorming result with no chest pain, no changes on the ECG and a normal blood pressure response, the patient may be immortal! Conversely, if the patient collapses in a heap after thirty seconds on the treadmill with the ECG trace waving around all over the place or a drop in blood pressure, the surgeon should start sharpening the knives.

In between these two extremes are the difficult patients who do quite well on the treadmill but perhaps not well enough. No one really knows where the cut-off point should be for when surgery should prevail over tablets. The treadmill test is far from perfect so much research has gone into using the radioactive scan techniques to look at the heart during exercise.

To summarise briefly, if there are multiple areas where the radioactive chemical does not get taken up, this would suggest that surgery is preferable to tablets. In order for research like this to be meaningful one has to study many patients and, with the help of some black magic and statisticians, it is possible to show differences that are scientifically acceptable between groups of patients who will do well without surgery and those that won't. The great difficulty for the doctor sitting in front of a patient is how to apply that information to the individual.

Supposing a very good piece of research shows that 70 per cent of patients with a particular pattern on the treadmill test or the thallium scan do better with surgery than with tablets, this means that 30 per cent of patients won't behave like that. All the specialist can do when recommending treatment to the individual in front of him is to apply the law of 'balance of probabilities'. The doctor has little way of knowing whether his patient falls into the 70 per cent group or the 30 per cent group but on the balance of probabilities the patient will do better with surgery than without. So, if you are seeing a heart specialist who strongly recommends that you have something done to your arteries even though you may not have terrible symptoms you may now understand why. Even with the most sophisticated tests though, we have to accept the unpredictability of nature and that biological tissue such as coronary arteries may cause problems that could never be foreseen.

A NATIONAL LOTTERY

Recently, some astonishing information was published by a working party commissioned by the government to look into the access and availability of balloon treatment and coronary by-pass operations around the UK. The results provided information that the government would rather not have heard.

Four health regions were picked out for study. These were South East Thames, East Anglia, Manchester and Glasgow. The results showed that there were up to 600 per cent variations in the likelihood of people receiving treatment, depending upon where they lived. Those who lived close to a major heart centre had a better deal than those who lived a long way away, and in the parts of the country where there was not a heart specialist the treatment rates were lowest.

The information shows what a lottery health care is, and it supports the impression of most heart specialists that there is a large untapped population who just aren't getting into the system. We clearly can't rely on government to increase spending on health care and when the medical profession shouts for a larger slice of the national cake it is just seen as another vested interest group screaming for more precious resources.

If we look at the number of procedures per million that are carried out and compare them with those of our European partners we can see how we fare. Britain has one of the highest incidences of death from heart disease in Europe, yet our record of by-pass operations (371 per million of the population in 1993) is substantially lower than those carried out in Austria, Belgium, Finland, Germany, Iceland, Holland, Sweden and Switzerland. We were slightly ahead of Denmark, Italy, Spain and Portugal and a long way ahead of Bulgaria, Lithuania, Poland and Slovenia. For balloon angioplasty in 1993 we carried out 226 procedures per million of the population whereas Belgium and Germany carried out over 850, Holland over 750, Switzerland over 650 and Sweden over 400. We were at the same level as Denmark and a little bit ahead of Italy.

TREATMENTS FOR DISEASED VALVES

With valve disease the treatment options are much less complicated. We can leave the valve alone, try to crack open a narrowed valve with a balloon, let the surgeon repair it or put in a new one. With all this information I am giving about blocked pipes and valves you may think that your heart specialist and cardiac surgeon are no more than highly skilled plumbers – the difference being that plumbers earn more!

In Chapter 4 I covered the common valve conditions and explained some of the decision-making processes which we use to decide whose valve should be left alone and who should have an operation. When there is a narrowed mitral valve this can often be split open with a balloon without a major heart operation. Your doctor will discuss with you whether he thinks you should have a new valve and why.

Sometimes your symptoms will tell you that something is wrong, although symptoms can develop late and only after the heart muscle has become stretched and damaged.

Your doctor will monitor the pumping function carefully and if the heart muscle shows signs of being put under undue strain, an operation will be recommended even if you feel reasonably well. This is done to protect your heart muscle from the inevitable consequences of becoming tired out.

In cases of the illness called endocarditis, the specialist will monitor how the infection has responded to antibiotics, whether it is beginning to show signs of a severe leak because it is being destroyed by the infection, and whether there is a mass of infected tissue (vegetations) on the valve. All these factors will be taken into account when the specialist recommends surgery and its timing.

Types of replacement valve

If you are advised to have a new valve the main concern will be the sort of valve put in. There are two types, natural or tissue valves which may come from a cow or a pig which have been sterilised and mounted in a cloth ring, and metallic valves which have a variety of ingenious designs from a ball and cage to various sorts of disks. There are advantages and disadvantages to each.

The tissue valves are made of naturally occurring biological material and the valves don't tend to develop blood clots on them. The main advantage of these is that it is not necessary to take blood-thinning tablets (warfarin). The trouble with the tissue valves is that they are not nearly as long-lasting as the metal ones and we would hesitate to put one of these valves into a young person because the valve may wear out and become furred up or leaky over the next ten to fifteen years.

For some reason that we don't fully understand, animal valves last longer in the elderly and wear out more quickly in the young. By 'elderly' I don't mean someone over the

231

age of 90 – research has shown that an animal valve might last twenty years in a 65-year-old but only ten years in a 20-year-old.

Metal valves overcome this problem, but it is necessary for patients to take warfarin regularly to prevent clots occurring on the metal. The big dilemma is what to do when treating women of child-bearing age, because if a woman takes warfarin during pregnancy there is a small risk that the baby might develop abnormalities. If a woman of child-bearing age needs a new valve we must discuss the risks and benefits of taking warfarin and having a very long-lasting and durable valve versus the likelihood that with a pig or cow valve a second operation will be necessary at some stage.

Some commercially available valves have had a bad press and many people have become alarmed by reports of certain types of metal valve breaking. If you are worried that your valve might be one of these please do not hesitate to ask your specialist, who will nearly always be able to reassure you.

Patients with mitral valve disease often have the rhythm disturbance called atrial fibrillation. The major risk of this condition is that blood clots form, so if a patient has atrial fibrillation and needs to be on warfarin anyway it makes sense to have a metal valve.

Metal valves tend to be noisier than animal valves and some people find it rather odd at first to hear their heart clicking away and making a noise a bit like a ping-pong ball. The doctor may be able to count the pulse rate of a patient just by listening from the end of the bed and patients with noisy artificial heart valves will make pretty awful cat burglars and lousy spies!

Doctors never recommend heart surgery lightly and my own advice would be to opt for a long-lasting valve, rather than take the risk of having to have a second operation just to avoid the minor nuisance of having to take blood-thinning tablets. It really isn't worth it.

Whatever valve you and your surgeon decide on, the operation is likely to be very safe. The major factor which influences the risk of the operation is how well the heart is pumping and what the cause of the valve problem is. The patient who has had a damaged pump for a long time will have a higher risk than one whose pump is normal. An emergency operation because of a sudden tear in the valve or because it has been destroyed very quickly by infection will also be riskier than a planned operation.

With all technology used in medicine, unforeseen problems may arise ten years down the line, in spite of all the testing before a product is licensed. Newer and better valves are being developed all the time and the overwhelming majority of people who have an artificial heart valve have many years of trouble-free motoring.

Aftercare

The same precautions with regard to dental hygiene, and antibiotic cover for dental procedures and any operation involving the bowels, intestines or obstetrics, apply to heart valve surgery. Artificial valves can become infected just as easily as your own valves except that infection of an artificial valve is much more serious and harder to treat.

If you have an artificial heart valve and have an unexplained illness with a temperature, shivers and shakes, or are off your food, or start to lose weight and feel generally unwell, please see your doctor quickly. You must always be alert to the possibility of infection (endocarditis) on an artificial heart valve.

If you have a metal valve which is noisy and you detect any change in the noise the valve makes, please contact your doctor straight away because this might mean that the valve is not working properly. You may well pooh-pooh this idea but there was one famous case many years ago when a woman with a metal valve was brought in one evening with the complaint: 'I hope I'm not wasting your time doctor but my valve which normally goes "clickety click, clickety click" is now just going "click"!'

Knowing what sort of valve she had in, it took a very short time for her doctor to realise that she was absolutely right to be concerned and she had the valve changed straight away.

TREATMENT FOR DAMAGED HEARTS

In the case of a severely damaged heart, a family of drugs called ACE inhibitors have been shown to improve survival and most doctors are now tuned in to prescribing these drugs as soon as possible after a large heart attack. These drugs may help the healing process and they reduce the amount of work the heart has to do and may be given in combination with drugs to reduce the congestion of the lungs. These fluid-reducing drugs are known as diuretics, and make the kidneys produce large amounts of urine, so there is a smaller volume of blood circulating around our body and, therefore, less likelihood of the lungs becoming congested.

Attention is also paid to the levels of certain chemicals in the blood, particularly to potassium levels. If the potassium is low, this can predispose the heart to electrical instability and rhythm disorders. Sometimes patients may therefore be asked to take potassium supplements in the form of tablets, or to eat foods which are high in potassium, such as bananas and tomato juice.

A damaged heart is also prone to rhythm disorders even if the potassium level is normal. Sometimes specific rhythm-controlling drugs will be given. Many of these drugs have side-effects, and great care goes into choosing which drug is right for individual patients. For example, people who have asthma or wheezing cannot take beta-blockers, because they make the wheezing worse. These and other drugs can further weaken the pumping function of the heart and, therefore, cannot be used. Some drugs cause blurred vision and a dry mouth and, in elderly men, difficulty in passing urine.

Often we are left with only one or two drugs which we can give, and the most powerful of these is called *amiodarone*. This is cardiac Domestos! It kills 99 per cent of all household rhythm disturbances! The trade-off is that side-effects are quite common, and careful monitoring is essential. A side-effect which nearly everybody on this drug will experience is an itchy rash on areas of the skin exposed to strong sunlight. Even in Britain, the sun between April and October can provoke this. Patients on this drug should be aware that they must use protective barrier cream on exposed areas and wear a sun hat to keep the sun off their face. Sun worshippers may find this intolerable, but if you are given amiodarone, you will have to accept that your sunbathing days may be over. Now, if some of you reading this are on amiodarone, do not panic. Amiodarone is not only given to people with severely damaged hearts, but it may be given because other drugs fail, even when the pumping function of the heart is normal. It may also be given to patients with HCM who have dangerous rhythm disorders (see page 103).

If rhythm-controlling drugs fail, some sort of implantable device may be needed as described in Chapter 6.

Transplants

As you know, you cannot go out and buy a heart in the

235

same way you can buy an artificial heart valve or pace-maker. In order for a heart to become available, someone else has to suffer a fatal tragedy. The ethics of donating organs, organ donor cards, and the way that families are approached for permission to use the organs of their loved ones are beyond the scope of this book. Doctors have to handle this issue very delicately.

However it is handled the fact is that the supply of hearts is limited and it is not possible for everyone needing a heart transplant to get one. Doctors are put in the posi-tion of having to play God, and deciding who is assessed for a heart transplant and who is not. Age limits, family needs, the suitability of the patient to cope with the rigor-ous drug regime, and the intensive aftercare that goes with heart transplantation, are all taken into consideration. Perhaps as technology evolves, the artificial or mechanical heart will become more widely available. My own view is that the artificial heart is the way to go in the future, and that some sort of implantable pumping device with a system of valves and a battery that does not depend on an external power source, could be developed over the next ten years or so. Let us hope so.

The heart transplant operation, as performed by heart surgeons, is not technically very difficult. The main prob-lem is with rejection, where the body recognises the organ as being 'foreign' and tries to attack it. Drugs are used to try to suppress the immune system's response to the new organ, and these drugs are called *immuno-suppressive drugs*. People who have had transplants may have to undergo biopsies at regular intervals to see if there is evidence of rejection which would require their drugs to be increased. When the heart is transplanted the coronary arteries are transplanted as well, and the rejection process tends to lead to these arteries becoming furred up. We have not yet found the perfect way of dealing with this. Again, an artificial heart which did not need a blood supply would be the ideal solution.

There are a few experimental procedures which have been used as alternatives to heart transplants. These include using one of the big muscles at the back and moving it to wrap around the heart and trying to 'train' the muscle to help the heart along. There are also temporary 'assist' devices which can be used in patients who are really ill to keep them going until a donor heart becomes available. These procedures are not widely used and the success rate has not been terrific.

I hope I have managed to convince you that your heart specialist will not select a treatment for you in the same way as score draws on a football coupon. The decision for any individual patient is based upon a broad knowledge of the scientific evidence available plus the invaluable bank of clinical experience which the specialist will have built up over the years.

11

BACK ON DRY LAND
LIFE AFTER THE KNIFE

BACK TO WORK?

It is usually obvious when someone is fit to go back to work. I have one patient, again a rabbi, who is an endless source of jokes but who had rather a rough time after his by-pass operation. I knew he was finally cured when his outpatient interview went like this:

ME: Now, do you have any questions about your medications?

RABBI: Only this. How many aspirins should I be taking?

ME: Two small tablets a day

RABBI: Good. If Moses had two tablets then so shall I.

ME: How much exercise are you doing?

RABBI: Not a lot, but then again you know that Moses never won a marathon.

ME: Sorry?

RABBI: Yes. The Bible says 'and Moses came forth'.

ME: Yes. I don't suppose you do any other exercise.

RABBI: You must be joking. But you know that Joseph (he of the multi-coloured coat) was a tennis player.

ME: Really?

RABBI: Yes. The Bible says 'and Joseph served in Pharaoh's court'.

Oy!

We encourage people to walk as much as possible to help the circulation in the legs back to normal and to aid general fitness. It is much easier to convalesce from heart surgery in the spring or the summer than in the cold winter months, but unfortunately we can't choose when our heart operations are necessary. Patients should usually be encouraged to get out and walk once they are discharged from hospital, start activities such as swimming after a few weeks, but not hurl themselves back into competitive games like squash! Patients may not drive immediately after a heart operation – this is largely to protect the breast bone – but after six weeks they can drive, swim and start lifting. Patients who hold HGV licences or drive buses, fire-engines or taxi-cabs have to satisfy strict criteria laid down by the licensing authorities that they are medically fit to drive before they can resume work. Some people get back to work quicker than others. A job which is home- or desk-based and doesn't involve too much commuting will be easier to return to quickly than a job which involves a lot of travelling or heavy lifting.

The issues of mental approach and lifestyle need serious contemplation. While we are young and healthy we set ourselves goals for the future, the pot of gold at the end of the rainbow. We work harder and harder, aiming to better ourselves for the new car, the holiday abroad or the stereo television. Before we know it we are well and truly stuck on the treadmill. As the rewards in life come flooding in, our egos and our wallets may feel the benefits, but at what cost to our coronary arteries?

At a certain point in our lives we tend to take stock and

think about what we have achieved and what our goals are for the next ten to fifteen years. Leaving home at six o'clock in the morning and getting back at nine thirty at night, and bringing work home at weekends may have all the hallmarks of success but there are quality-of-life issues which need to be addressed as well. It only takes illness or the death of a close friend, relative or colleague to make us realise that working excessively hard now in order to have a comfortable retirement may not always be a sensible approach. None of us is immortal although we always fall into the trap of assuming that heart attacks or death from other illnesses happen to other people, never to us.

Many people have commented on a subtle shift which is taking place both in Europe and in the United States in what people want from their lives. The Americans, as is their wont, have coined the phrase 'down reaching' or 'down shifting', where people with highly successful and demanding careers have deliberately chosen to change their way of life and accept a lower income and a smaller house in exchange for more personal freedom and time to enjoy some of the non-commercial things in life.

On this side of the Atlantic we are used to disillusioned politicians wishing to 'spend more time with their families' – and sometimes they really mean it – but it often takes a major event such as a heart attack to force people to examine how they spend their time.

Although most people get back to normal after a heart attack or heart surgery, people perceive their work environment as having contributed to their illness in the first place. Hard work and stress on their own are unlikely to cause arteries to fur up but the stress associated with certain jobs may lead to increased smoking, high blood pleasure, a sedentary lifestyle and an unhealthy diet. We have to ask ourselves whether it is reasonable to expect people who are medically well after a heart attack or a heart operation to return to the environment in which they first became ill. This is a major issue for many people and there are many financial implications for the breadwinner of the family as well as for insurance companies who pay out sickness benefit or permanent health insurance if someone is unfit to return to work. Policies may pay you an income while you are medically unfit but will not go on paying you if you are psychologically unable to get back to work.

We have here a conflict of interest between employers and insurers. A company may expect its sales director to drive around 60,000 miles a year, if not more, fly off round the world at regular intervals and be a slave to his job. A sales director, having had a heart attack may be medically quite well but psychologically may feel quite unable to bring the same gusto to the job as before the attack. Such a person is therefore not medically but psychologically disabled.

The company may not want an individual who is not firing on all cylinders back at work, and the individual may tremble at the thought of resuming the former lifestyle. Businesses and corporations which have paid large premiums for sickness or permanent health insurance may look to the insuring agencies to pay their sales director a generous sum on the basis of disablement. The insurance company will ask the doctor for supporting medical evidence and the patient's GP will almost always take the side of the patient and express the view that someone who has had a heart attack or a heart operation cannot be reasonably expected to go back to such a high-pressured job. If the patient has been under the care of a heart specialist locally it is almost certain that this specialist will also take the side of the patient and advocate early retirement. The insurance company may therefore ask for an independent medical opinion.

The issue is not whether or not the individual had a

heart attack but whether he or she is medically fit to go back to work. Insurance policies differ. Some specify that the patient must be unfit to resume the original job and some specify he or she must be unfit to resume any employment. The role of the independent specialist is to make sure, as far as possible, that this is not a case of *plumbum oscillans.* (This is not jargon – it is Latin for lead swinging!)

The insurance industry has yet to come to terms with the fact that you don't have to be clutching your chest with pain or gasping for breath in order to be medically unfit to return to your previous employment. At the same time the insured individual must realise that an insurance company cannot be expected to fork out large sums of money so that the client can spend five days a week on the golf course enjoying the life of Riley. This is a grey area, where each case needs to be assessed on its merits.

Although in some cases a patient may not be able to go back to the same job as before, people who have had a heart attack or heart surgery should not regard themselves as being invalids and should be encouraged to lead a productive life. This is less applicable to people who have a heart attack or operation in their early or mid fifties. Studies have shown that return to work patterns after balloon treatment or by-pass surgery are disappointing. We don't go around operating on people in order that they should be considered invalids afterwards, and part of the recovery from a heart attack or heart operation would, in an ideal world, involve psychological counselling and rehabilitation.

The lack of cardiac rehabilitation (where patients are given support and advice on their return to work) may be one of the reasons why return to work patterns are not as high as we would like. However, most heart specialists are so busy trying to cope with acutely ill patients that they don't have the time to give the counselling many people require. Patients do need help to adopt the right mental approach and I cannot overstate that the fact that a zipper down the front of the chest is not a disabled label. On the contrary, on the west coast of the United States the open heart surgery zipper is something of a status symbol!

Some patients revel in their heart illness. They use it as a topic of conversation at dinner parties and like to dramatise their condition. These patients never *go* to hospital but are *rushed* to hospital; never see *a* specialist but *the top* specialist; never have a *heart attack* but a *massive heart attack*; never have *a by-pass* but a *quadruple by-pass*.

PRIMARY PREVENTION

Perversely, the ultimate goal of heart specialists who spend most of their time dealing with diseases caused by furred-up and blocked arteries is to put themselves out of business. It is the job of the specialist and the teams of nurses, dietitians and those who work on rehabilitation programmes, not only to perform high-technology procedures but to try to prevent people getting the diseases in the first place. This 'primary prevention' is easier said than done.

Much research is now going on into identifying the genes which are responsible for premature coronary disease, particularly in patients with high cholesterol levels that run in families. Many of these people have no preventable risk factors and one hopes that one of the beneficial uses of the controversial technique of genetic engineering might be to solve this difficult problem, along with other non self-inflicted diseases such as diabetes.

Some years ago an eminent American cardiologist published a wonderful description of the ideal coronary risk-free male: 'An effeminate municipal worker or embalmer, completely lacking in physical or mental alertness and without drive, ambition or competitive spirit, who has never attempted to meet a deadline of any kind. A man with poor appetite, subsisting on fruits and vegetables laced with corn and whale oil, detesting tobacco, spurning ownership of radio, tv or motor car, with full head of hair and scrawny and unathletic in appearance, yet constantly straining his puny muscles by exercise; low in income, blood pressure, blood sugar and cholesterol ... who has been taking long term anti-coagulant therapy ever since his prophylactic castration.' (Henry Blackburn quoting Gordon Myers of Boston in *American Journal of Cardiology* July 1986.)

If genetic engineering produces males like this the human race is destined for extinction. Even if this male had not had a castration no woman in her right mind would find him attractive enough to want to have his child! The idea of a genetically engineered, medically perfect human race is horrific but it is not beyond the bounds of possibility that at some time in the future certain forms of coronary disease could be genetically treated.

More practically, we cannot force people to eat a healthy diet, to take regular exercise, not to start smoking or become overweight. What we can and must do is to keep hammering home the message that by setting our children off on the correct path to good habits we can minimise their risk for the future.

I am not suggesting that parents should deny their children sweets or chocolates but we are doing them no favours by allowing them to indulge in mega-burgers and big fat wizard waffles to their heart's delight (or rather, torture). If parents set their children a bad example by smoking around the house then we must not be surprised if this habit is perpetuated through the generations. In the scale of medical misery, more long-term harm is done by regular heavy smoking than by the occasional use of illegal soft drugs. This should not be misinterpreted to assume that I am in favour of legalising soft drugs, I am merely pointing out the perverse nature of our publicity machines which focus so much on one aspect while ignoring the other.

Still, working on the promise that prevention is better than cure, I now invite you to go through the following questionnaire.

1   Are you:
    A   A teenager?
    B   A woman?
    C   A man?
    D   None of the above?
    E   A wrinkled, grey-haired smoking man under the age of 55 or a bald, deaf, wig-wearing woman from the north of England?

2   When did you/will you give up smoking?
    A   Twenty years ago
    B   Five years ago
    C   This morning
    D   Tomorrow
    E   Never, never, never

3   Your favourite meal is:
    A   Corn, vegetables and fruit laced with whale oil
    B   Pasta, fresh tomatoes and fruit
    C   Fish cooked in batter with chips and tomato sauce
    D   A plate of cream cakes
    E   Three eggs, two rashers of bacon and fried bread, dipped in lard

4   When you have the urge to exercise do you:

A   Go for a brisk walk or a swim?

B   Pull your stomach muscles in and kid yourself you don't need the exercise?

C   Lift up the TV guide twenty times with each arm?

D   Lie down until the urge to exercise passes?

E   Never have the urge so not applicable?

5   **Five of your close male relatives have had heart attacks and you have high cholesterol. Do you:**

A   Ask to go onto cholesterol-lowering drugs?

B   Work hard at your diet and weight?

C   Cut out one or two eggs per week?

D   Change your name by deed poll or have a sex change if you are a man?

E   Shrug your shoulders and console yourself with a cigarette?

6   **You have a work deadline which is virtually impossible but your promotion prospects depend on it. The deadline coincides with your wedding anniversary. Do you:**

A   Resign yourself to not achieving promotion, tear up the brochure for a new Porsche and go out to dinner with your spouse?

B   Ask for an attractive assistant of the appropriate gender?

C   Mildly protest to your boss but do your best and crack open a a bottle of bubbly with your spouse during a half-hour break from work?

D   Cancel the wedding anniversary celebrations, stock up with coffee and cigarettes and tell your spouse not to expect you?

E   Work yourself into a hot sweaty lather, develop palpitations, insomnia and nausea?

7   **You are 45 years old and at a health screening you
    are told you are 3 stone overweight and have high
    blood pressure. Do you:**

    A   Feel shaken and resolve to slim down and have
    your blood pressure monitored monthly?

    B   Take blood pressure pills and cut out potatoes
    and biscuits?

    C   Agree reluctantly to take blood pressure pills
    and ignore your weight?

    D   Reply that your grandmother had high blood
    pressure and lived to the age of 90 and that your
    spouse likes a bit of flesh to grab?

    E   Go on a complete starvation diet and take up
    competitive squash with a 20-year-old?

8   **You have had a tightness in your chest while walk-
    ing to the station on a cold morning. Do you:**

    A   Badger your GP until you get an early appoint-
    ment?

    B   Ring up your golf partner who is a gynaecologist
    and seek advice?

    C   Think about phoning the doctor but don't want
    to make too much of a fuss?

    D   Blame it on the cold air and just wear a scarf next
    time?

    E   Put it down to last night's curry and reach for
    the Milk of Magnesia?

How did you score?

Mainly As
You clearly take your health very seriously, you have a sensible attitude to life and if you are unlucky enough to get
heart disease you will probably recognise the symptoms

and seek medical help.

Mainly Bs
You probably think that you are not really at risk from heart trouble and make a reluctant attempt to eat and work sensibly. You probably like to stay away from doctors unless you meet them on the golf course.

Mainly Cs
You have a head-in-the-sand attitude to health. The road to Hades is paved with good intentions and you would probably like someone to wave a magic wand and make all your risk factors go away. You certainly could never be accused of bothering your doctor too much.

Mainly Ds
Publicity on health promotion obviously whistles past you like the winter winds. You are probably well down the road to ruin and you almost certainly fail to recognise a heart attack if it jumped up and went 'boo'.

Mainly Es
Oh dear. Please go back to the beginning and read the book again from cover to cover. It would be sensible for you to book your appointment with a heart specialist now.

INDEX